Field Guide to the Eyes

Field Guide to the Eyes

Jonathan D. Trobe, M.D.
Director of Ophthalmology and Neurology
Kellogg Eye Center
Department of Ophthalmology and Visual Science
University of Michigan
Ann Arbor, Michigan

Richard E. Hackel, M.A., C.R.A.
Director of Ophthalmic Photography
Kellogg Eye Center
Department of Ophthalmology and Visual Science
University of Michigan
Ann Arbor, Michigan

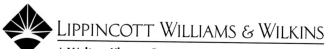

LIPPINCOTT WILLIAMS & WILKINS
A **Wolters Kluwer** Company

Philadelphia · Baltimore · New York · London
Buenos Aires · Hong Kong · Sydney · Tokyo

Acquisitions Editor: Richard Winters
Development Editor: Pamela Sutton
Production Editor: Deirdre Marino
Manufacturing Manager: Colin Warnock
Compositor: Maryland Composition
Printer: Quebecor World Color

© 2002 by LIPPINCOTT WILLIAMS & WILKINS
530 Walnut Street
Philadelphia, PA 19106 USA
LWW.com

Library of Congress Cataloging-in-Publicaton Data

Trobe, Jonathan D., 1943–
    Field guide to the eyes / Jonathan D. Trobe, Richard E. Hackel.
        p. ; cm.
    Includes index.
    ISBN 0-7817-3168-2
    1. Eye—Diseases—Handbooks, manuals, etc. 2. Eye—Diseases—Diagnosis. 3. Eye—Diseases—Atlases. I. Hackel, Richard E. II. Title.
    [DNLM: 1. Eye Diseases—diagnosis—Handbooks. 2. Eye Diseases—therapy—Handbooks. WW 39 T843f2002]
    RE48.9 .T76 2002
    617.7—dc21
                                                              2001050626

10 9 8 7 6 5 4 3 2 1

Contents

Contents

III. Iris, Lens, and Vitreous

IV: Retina and Optic Nerve

Appendices

Preface

This book is designed to be the fastest, most practical way to help the reader identify and screen for eye problems. Recognizing eye problems is much like recognizing birds, so we have followed the example of the ornithologist James Audubon, who fashioned his guidebooks to the birds in this way. You will find one (or sometimes two or three) classic photographs for each entity fitted with the answers to six questions: What is it? What does it look like? What else looks like it? How do you diagnose? How do you manage? What is the outcome? We have tried to distinguish your role as primary care physician from that of the ophthalmologist. For example, we tell you when and how quickly to refer, when to treat, and when to leave the problem alone. In the appendices, you will encounter illustrated "how to's" about screening for eye problems and handling common eye manifestations. The book concludes with a synopsis of commonly used ophthalmic medications.

Acknowledgments

Thanks to Csaba Martonyi, C.R.A, F.O.P.S, Sally Stanley, C.R.A, and Robert Prusak, C.R.A, for photographs culled from a vast collection taken over 30 years of ophthalmic photography at the Kellogg Eye Center, University of Michigan; to M. Madison Slusher, M.D., Chairman of the Wake Forest University Eye Center in Winston-Salem, and Marshall E. Tyler, C.R.A, F.O.P.S for use of photographs; and to Howard Schatz, M.D., for guidance and inspiration.

Field Guide to the Eyes

Stye

WHAT IS IT?

Also called a chalazion or hordeolum, it is an acute sterile inflammation of the meibomian sebaceous glands of the lid margin. The orifices of the glands become plugged, sebum escapes into neighboring lid tissue, and a sterile foreign body reaction creates the inflammation.

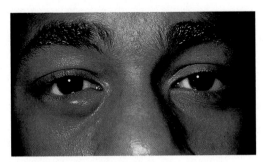

FIGURE 1. Stye. Medial right lower lid is swollen and red.

WHAT DOES IT LOOK LIKE?

A painful, tender, reddish subcutaneous mound on the eyelid, typically near its margin. At times the surrounding lid is so swollen it is hard to locate the mass.

WHAT ELSE LOOKS LIKE IT?

Orbital cellulitis and dacryocystitis. But orbital cellulitis is nonfocal, and both lids are usually swollen and tight. Dacryocystitis is always located in the medial lower lid, away from the margin; purulent material may emerge from the lower punctum on compression of the lacrimal sac.

HOW DO YOU DIAGNOSE?

By clinical signs.

HOW DO YOU MANAGE?

Advise the patient to apply warm compresses twice daily. Antimicrobial or corticosteroid treatment is not indicated.

WHAT IS THE OUTCOME?

The inflammation usually resolves within a week. Sometimes a painless mound persists from reparative scarring. Surgical excision may then be necessary. If chronic blepharitis is present, it may require separate treatment (see Chapter 2). Refer only if the mass continues to grow or fails to disappear after several weeks. An enlarging lid mass may be a sebaceous carcinoma.

Blepharitis

WHAT IS IT?

A chronic sterile or staphylococcal inflammation of the skin, cilia follicles, meibomian, or accessory glands of the eyelids.

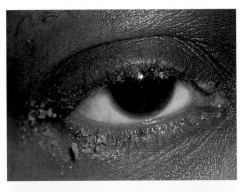

A

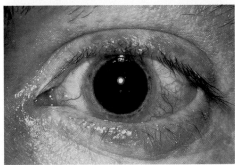

B

FIGURE 1. Blepharitis. **A:** Lid margins encrusted with seborrheic debris. **B:** Lid margins diffusely and irregularly swollen and red.

WHAT DOES IT LOOK LIKE?

Patients complain of a gritty, burning sensation in their eyes, especially on awakening. Lid margins are slightly and diffusely swollen, hyperemic, and irregular. Lashes are sometimes encrusted with seborrheic debris. These findings may be very subtle, especially without the help of a slit lamp biomicroscope. The conjunctiva may be mildly hyperemic. The face and scalp may show signs of rosacea or hyperkeratotic dermatitis.

WHAT ELSE LOOKS LIKE IT?

Chronic mild conjunctivitis and keratitis. But conjunctivitis fails to produce the characteristic lid signs, and keratitis should show abnormalities highlighted with a slit lamp.

HOW DO YOU DIAGNOSE?

By clinical signs.

HOW DO YOU MANAGE?

Have the patient perform lid margin scrubs as follows:

1. Place a warm washcloth over the closed lids for 5 minutes to soften crusts.
2. Fill a container with 3 oz of warm water and add 3 drops of baby shampoo (any brand). Moisten a cotton-tipped applicator in the solution and use it to scrub the closed lids. Brush off lid margin debris with the applicator.
3. If the lid scrubs are not effective within 4 weeks, prescribe bacitracin or erythromycin ointment nightly.
4. If this does not work, prescribe oral tetracycline 0.5 to 1 g/day in four doses or doxycycline 50 to 100 mg once or twice daily (except in pregnancy and in children aged 12 years or less).

WHAT IS THE OUTCOME?

Blepharitis usually responds to one or more of these measures within weeks but often recurs when treatment is stopped. Retreatment usually works. Refer recalcitrant cases.

CHAPTER 3

Ectropion

WHAT IS IT?

An eversion of the lower lid so that it no longer lies in apposition to the surface of the eye. It may be congenital or acquired. Most cases are acquired and are caused by involutional laxity. Seventh cranial nerve palsy and inflammation, trauma, or resection of cheek skin can also cause ectropion.

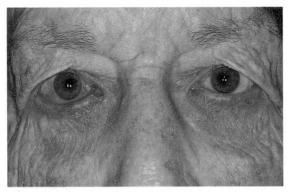

FIGURE 1. Ectropion. Right lower lid is everted, and its margin is not apposed to the eye.

WHAT DOES IT LOOK LIKE?

The patient complains of eye irritation and tearing. The lower lid hangs down and away from the eye so that the lower conjunctiva becomes much too exposed. With the lid displaced from the eye surface, tears do not make their way to the punctum and instead pour out onto the cheek. The conjunctiva may be hyperemic, and the lower corneal epithelium may show punctate staining from drying.

WHAT ELSE LOOKS LIKE IT?

Nothing.

HOW DO YOU DIAGNOSE?

By clinical signs.

HOW DO YOU MANAGE?

If the ectropion is not severe, the patient has no complaints, and the corneal surface is intact, no treatment is needed. For moderate ectropion, a nightly application of sterile ointment may be enough. If not, a surgical tightening procedure is indicated.

WHAT IS THE OUTCOME?

Surgical lid tightening is usually successful for involutional laxity. But if lower lid or cheek skin has been lost or scarred, complicated grafting may be necessary.

CHAPTER 4

Entropion

WHAT IS IT?

An inversion of the upper or lower lid so that its margin points toward the eye. The biggest problem is that the lashes are now aimed inward and may abrade the corneal surface. The usual cause of lower lid entropion is involutional lid laxity. Upper lid entropion usually results from scarring after inflammation, trauma, or recent eye or periocular surgery.

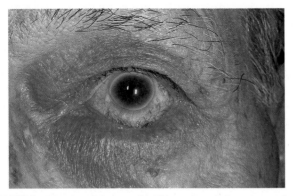

FIGURE 1. Entropion, right lower lid. Lid margin curls in on the eye, its lashes poking the cornea.

WHAT DOES IT LOOK LIKE?

The patient complains of a foreign body sensation, photophobia, and sometimes blurred vision from lash abrasion of the corneal surface. The affected cornea may stain with fluorescein. The lid margin curls inward, and the lashes point toward the cornea.

WHAT ELSE LOOKS LIKE IT?

Nothing.

HOW DO YOU DIAGNOSE?

By clinical signs.

HOW DO YOU MANAGE?

Surgical eversion of the lid is the only solution.

WHAT IS THE OUTCOME?

Surgery to evert the lid is usually successful but may be complicated.

CHAPTER 5
Lid Neoplasm

WHAT IS IT?

A tumor of the lid usually caused by basal or squamous cell carcinoma and rarely by sebaceous cell carcinoma.

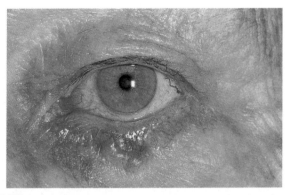

FIGURE 1. Basal cell carcinoma. A crater depression, as seen here, is common. Many tumors are dome-shaped.

WHAT DOES IT LOOK LIKE?

A firm, nontender lump on the lid. It enlarges but usually very slowly. The lid margin may be distorted, and any shape or color is possible. The surface may be ulcerated.

WHAT ELSE LOOKS LIKE IT?

Warts, nevi, keratoses, keratoacanthomas, epidermal and sebaceous inclusion cysts, papillomas, and molluscum contagiosum.

HOW DO YOU DIAGNOSE?

By clinical signs. But neoplasms cannot be distinguished from benign growths by appearance alone. Biopsy is the only way to be sure.

HOW DO YOU MANAGE?

Biopsy any new, growing, or suspicious lesion. Malignancies are treated surgically with the aim of having tumor-free margins. Skin grafts and flaps may be necessary when wide excision is required. Radiation and cryotherapy are alternative treatment methods, particularly when surgery cannot provide acceptable functional or cosmetic results. Radiation may cause a dry eye.

WHAT IS THE OUTCOME?

Depends on the pathology and its extent. Small basal cell cancers can usually be cured with surgery that does not cause lingering functional or cosmetic problems. Squamous carcinoma is notorious for spreading intracranially along sensory nerves even from a superficially small mass. Early diagnosis leads to better results.

CHAPTER 6
Herpes Zoster Ophthalmicus

WHAT IS IT?

Blistering dermatitis in the first division of the trigeminal nerve caused by herpes zoster. The virus is usually acquired during a varicella (chicken pox) infection in childhood and lies dormant in the trigeminal ganglion. Aging, stress, or illness causes it to spread retrograde down nerves supplying trigeminal dermatomes.

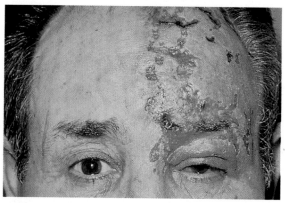

FIGURE 1. Trigeminal herpes zoster dermatitis. Note that the vesicles do not extend across the midforehead line.

WHAT DOES IT LOOK LIKE?

A painful, weepy crop of blisters on inflamed skin limited to the first trigeminal division—the forehead, upper eyelid, and sometimes the nose. If the tip of the nose is involved, chances are the cornea or uveal tract is also inflamed. If so, the conjunctiva will be hyperemic and biomicroscopy will show signs of keratitis or uveitis.

WHAT ELSE LOOKS LIKE IT?

Herpes simplex dermatitis, but it is usually not so strictly confined to a trigeminal division.

HOW DO YOU DIAGNOSE?

By clinical signs. Biopsy of skin lesions may be useful in confirming the diagnosis, but clinical signs are usually specific enough.

HOW DO YOU MANAGE?

Treat immunocompetent patients with oral acyclovir (800 mg 5×/day) or its derivatives famciclovir (500 mg t.i.d.) and valacyclovir (1 g t.i.d.) for 7 to 10 days. Immunocompromised hosts should receive intravenous acyclovir (5 to 10 mg/kg q8h for 7 to 10 days). Acyclovir and its derivative agents reduce viral dissemination and the chances of postherpetic neuralgia, but they do not hasten resolution. Corticosteroid treatment is not effective in reducing the chances of postherpetic neuralgia and may promote dissemination. Topical corticosteroids are used to treat keratitis and uveitis.

WHAT IS THE OUTCOME?

The skin lesions heal within weeks but sometimes leave scars. The major problem is lingering pain in the trigeminal distribution—postherpetic neuralgia. It occurs in more than 70% of patients older than age 60, despite acyclovir treatment of the acute lesions. Management, rarely totally palliative, involves tricyclic antidepressants (amitriptyline, nortryptiline, doxepin), topical anesthetics and capsaicin, oral opioids and nonsteroidal antiinflammatory drugs (NSAIDs), and transcutaneous electrical nerve stimulation (TENS), as well as somatic and sympatholytic nerve blocks.

Herpes zoster keratitis and uveitis may also be chronic and must be managed by an ophthalmologist.

CHAPTER 7

Contact Dermatoconjunctivitis

WHAT IS IT?

An allergic reaction of periocular skin and conjunctiva to contact with topical ocular medications or lid cosmetics. The major offenders contain neomycin.

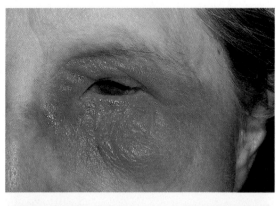

A

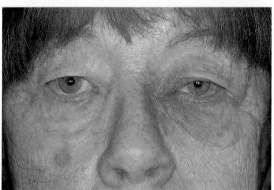

B

FIGURE 1. Contact dermatitis of eyelids. **A:** Severe eczematous redness and thickening of periocular skin. **B:** A mild case shows minimal lid inflammation.

WHAT DOES IT LOOK LIKE?

Eczematous redness and induration of the lid and cheek skin. The conjunctiva is often hyperemic (see Chapter 31 on chemical conjunctivitis).

WHAT ELSE LOOKS LIKE IT?

Other eczematous dermatitides, but they rarely produce findings limited to the periocular regions.

HOW DO YOU DIAGNOSE?

By learning that the patient has recently begun instilling an ocular medication or using a different lid cosmetic.

HOW DO YOU MANAGE?

By eliminating the offending agent.

WHAT IS THE OUTCOME?

Resolution is prompt and complete within days.

CHAPTER 8
Seventh Cranial Nerve Palsy

WHAT IS IT?

Paralysis of the seventh cranial nerve, which weakens the subcutaneous facial muscles, including the orbicularis oculi. Weakness of this muscle interferes with lid closure and causes the lower lid to droop down and away from the eye. As a result, the exposed lower cornea may become dry, ulcerated, and sometimes infected.

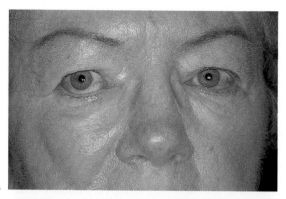

A

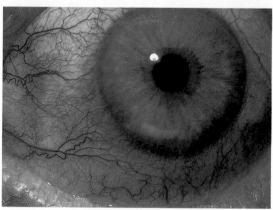

B

FIGURE 1. Seventh cranial nerve palsy. **A:** Depression of the right lower lid exposes the lower cornea and conjunctiva. **B:** Fluorescein staining discloses a green patch, a sign of dry, denuded corneal epithelium.

The usual cause of the palsy is a presumed viral infection (Bell's palsy), although trauma, infarct, and tumor may rarely be responsible. Eye exposure is not a problem from facial paralysis induced by an upper motor neuron seventh cranial nerve palsy (hemispheric stroke or tumor) because the upper face is rarely affected.

WHAT DOES IT LOOK LIKE?

The affected side of the face sags, and its subcutaneous muscles do not contract normally during smiling, blinking, and forehead wrinkling. Unlike a normal lower lid, which lies against the bottom edge of the cornea, a palsied lid droops and exposes the lower conjunctiva. With forced lid closure, the eye remains visible. If the cornea is substantially exposed, the patient will complain of eye pain and photophobia. Topical instillation of fluorescein stains green the areas of corneal epithelial denudation.

WHAT ELSE LOOKS LIKE IT?

Nothing.

HOW DO YOU DIAGNOSE?

By noting facial asymmetry and reduced contractions of the facial muscles on the affected side. Lower motor neuron facial palsy weakens the brow and periocular muscles; upper motor neuron facial palsy does not.

HOW DO YOU MANAGE?

There are two issues: (a) managing the facial palsy and (b) protecting the eye. If the palsy cannot be attributed to a viral cause, neurodiagnostic studies must be performed. For the facial palsy, a 7-day course of tapered oral corticosteroid treatment has been customary but is of unproved efficacy.

If the eye is exposed, prescribe over-the-counter artificial tears (any brand) to be instilled hourly during the day. If standard tears are not enough, prescribe viscous formulations such as carboxymethylcellulose sodium 0.5% (Refresh Plus) or 1% (Celluvisc). Prescribe petrolatum ophthalmic ointment to be deposited before bedtime in the lower conjunctival cul-de-sac. Patching is problematic because if the lids do not close, the patch will abrade the cornea. If lubrication does not protect the cornea, the patient may have to undergo suture apposition of the lids (tarsorrhaphy).

WHAT IS THE OUTCOME?

Depends on the degree of exposure and the duration of the palsy. Mild cases can usually be managed medically; severe palsies require tarsorrhaphy. The patient's symptoms (pain, photophobia, and blurred vision) and conjunctival hyperemia are usually reliable guides of how well the cornea is tolerating the exposure, except in patients who also have lesions of the trigeminal nerve and have lost corneal sensation.

CHAPTER 9
Xanthelasma

WHAT IS IT?

Xanthelasma are yellow-ochre mounds in the eyelids, usually located around the medial skin creases. Pathologically, they consist of collections of dermal perivascular lipid-filled macrophages and are often associated with Type II or III hyperlipoproteinemias.

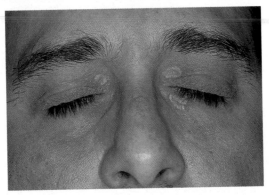

FIGURE 1. Eyelid xanthelasma. Yellow-brown plaques centered in medial eyelid skin folds represent lipid deposition in a patient with hyperlipidemia.

WHAT DOES IT LOOK LIKE?

Raised, yellow-ochre, oval or rectangular patches within the loose skin of the medial eyelids.

WHAT ELSE LOOKS LIKE IT?

Nothing.

HOW DO YOU DIAGNOSE?

Appearance alone is diagnostic; biopsy is confirmatory.

HOW DO YOU MANAGE?

By lowering elevated serum lipids. If that does not work, surgical excision is an option.

WHAT IS THE OUTCOME?

The lesions usually disappear if serum lipids normalize. If not, surgical excision may eliminate them, although they often return. Repeated excision may eventually work but can cause scarring and lid deformity.

CHAPTER 10
Capillary Hemangioma

WHAT IS IT?

A benign tumor of subcutaneous capillaries usually affecting the upper lid and sometimes the orbit of infants. It may be present at birth but usually develops weeks to months later, often enlarging so much that the lid occludes the eye. It reaches maximum size by 12 months and in-

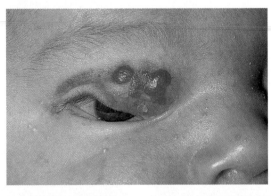

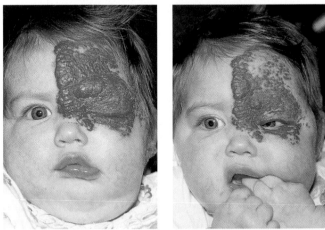

FIGURE 1. Capillary hemangioma. **A:** Vascular tumor causes ptosis. **B:** Massive capillary hemangioma of the upper face causes complete ptosis. **C:** Two months after intralesional triamcinolone injection, the lesion has shrunk enough so that the eye is visible.

volutes at age 4 to 6 years. The major concerns are a cosmetic blemish, fear of malignancy, and amblyopia.

WHAT DOES IT LOOK LIKE?

Raised, raspberry-like, dark-red clumps on the lid without surrounding inflammation.

WHAT ELSE LOOKS LIKE IT?

Nothing.

HOW DO YOU DIAGNOSE?

Appearance alone is diagnostic; biopsy is not necessary and causes heavy bleeding.

HOW DO YOU MANAGE?

Small lesions may be observed. Large masses that obstruct the visual axis and could cause amblyopia are treated by intralesional injection of triamcinolone.

WHAT IS THE OUTCOME?

Following intralesional injection, most lesions shrink dramatically within months to provide enough of an opening so that amblyopia does not occur. Even without treatment, the lesions disappear without a trace by age 6 to 7 years.

CHAPTER 11
Ptosis

WHAT IS IT?

Droopiness of the upper lid caused by paralysis of the third (oculomotor) cranial nerve, myasthenia gravis, the sympathetic nerve supply, a lid or orbital lesion, or senescent weakening of the levator tendon.

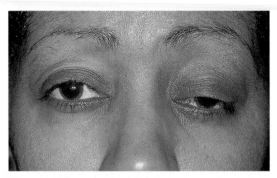

FIGURE 1. Ptosis. Left upper lid is droopy. The lesion may be in the levator palpebrae, in Müller's muscle, or in their innervations.

WHAT DOES IT LOOK LIKE?

The upper lid margin hangs too low, covering some or all of the cornea. The normal position of the upper lid varies greatly from one individual to another. However, a good guide is that the upper lid should not obscure more than 1 mm of the upper cornea. Unilateral ptosis is much easier to spot than bilateral ptosis because a normal lid is available for comparison.

WHAT ELSE LOOKS LIKE IT?

Dermatochalasis and blepharospasm. Dermatochalasis is a redundancy of upper lid skin, which flaps over the upper lid margin. If you lift this flap of skin, you will see that the upper lid margin is in the normal position. Blepharospasm is an involuntary contraction of the orbicularis oculi, tightening the palpebral fissure. Unlike ptosis, blepharospasm causes depression of the affected brow and elevation of the lower lid.

Sometimes ptosis is incorrectly diagnosed in one eye when the other eye has pathologic lid retraction (elevation). Also, an eye that is sunken in the orbit as the result of trauma may give the false impression of ptosis.

HOW DO YOU DIAGNOSE?

By noting that the upper lid covers more than 1 mm of the upper cornea. Look for features of third cranial nerve palsy (eye movement deficits, a dilated pupil), other signs of myasthenic weakness, sympathoparesis (a miotic pupil), or a lid or orbital mass.

HOW DO YOU MANAGE?

Depends on the diagnosis, which is difficult enough to warrant consultation with a specialist.

WHAT IS THE OUTCOME?

Depends on the diagnosis.

CHAPTER 12

Dermatochalasis

WHAT IS IT?

Redundant skin of the upper lid that hangs over the lid margin. It is usually caused by involutional loosening of skin, but may follow recurrent lid inflammation.

WHAT DOES IT LOOK LIKE?

The eye is hooded by overhanging upper lid skin. Sometimes the brow is also low because of loose forehead skin. But unlike the situation in ptosis or blepharospasm, the upper lid margin is in the normal position.

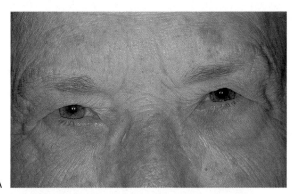

A

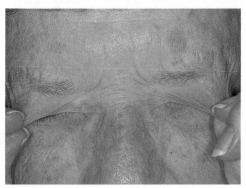

B

FIGURE 1. Dermatochalasis. **A:** Redundant upper lid skin hoods the eyes. **B:** Grabbing the skin reveals how much excess there is.

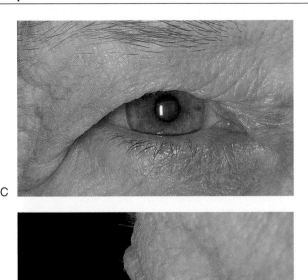

FIGURE 1. *Continued.* Hooding is even more evident in frontal (**C**) and side (**D**) close-up views.

Although it is usually a bilateral condition, it may be markedly asymmetric. Patients complain that their eyes feel heavy and that their view is blocked by an awning.

WHAT ELSE LOOKS LIKE IT?

Ptosis and blepharospasm. Ptosis is a droop of the upper lid margin. Blepharospasm is an episodic involuntary contraction of the orbicularis oculi, tightening the palpebral fissure.

HOW DO YOU DIAGNOSE?

By noting the upper lid skin redundancy that creates a flap overhanging the upper lid margin. You can lift the skin up to observe the normally positioned upper lid margin. Also note the commonly associated brow droop.

HOW DO YOU MANAGE?

If the condition is severe enough to be a cosmetic problem or to interfere with vision, the excess upper lid skin must be surgically excised. This procedure is often combined with a brow lift and removal of herniating orbital fat.

WHAT IS THE OUTCOME?

Well-performed surgery usually solves the problem, although repeat procedures are sometimes necessary.

CHAPTER 13

Blepharospasm

WHAT IS IT?

Episodic involuntary contraction of the orbicularis oculi. Usually bilateral and idiopathic (essential blepharospasm), it may be part of a parkinsonian disorder. Whether essential blepharospasm is a focal dystonic neurologic disorder or an expression of a psychiatric disorder remains unsettled. When blepharospasm is unilateral, it may be part of hemifacial spasm, a condition that results from irritation of the seventh cranial nerve by an aberrant vessel at the nerve's exit from the brainstem.

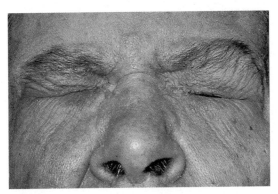

FIGURE 1. Blepharospasm. Patient forcefully and involuntarily closes her eyes.

WHAT DOES IT LOOK LIKE?

The patient reports an uncontrollable urge to close the eyes. The urge is often provoked by bright light or the emotional stress of interpersonal encounters. Contraction of the upper and lower lid (orbicularis) muscles narrows the palpebral fissure. If other facial muscles are involved, the face may be intermittently contorted or ridden by tics. The neurological exam is intact unless the patient has a parkinsonian condition.

WHAT ELSE LOOKS LIKE IT?

Nothing else produces such episodic contractions. Many patients are initially diagnosed as having keratitis (dry eye syndrome) because they appear to be complaining of photophobia. But patients with keratitis do not have such vigorous intermittent involuntary eyelid closure. Another misdiagnosis is focal seizure of the facial muscles.

HOW DO YOU DIAGNOSE?

By noting the episodic contractions of the facial (orbicularis) muscles in the absence of any ophthalmologic or neurologic abnormalities.

HOW DO YOU MANAGE?

If essential blepharospasm is provoked by anxiety, anxiolytic medications may be effective. If not, and the spasms are disruptive, subcutaneous botulinum toxin injections into the orbicularis oculi are often effective for periods of 1 to 6 months and are without adverse effects if done properly. If the blepharospasm is part of a parkinsonian disorder, treatment must be directed at the underlying problem. If the blepharospasm is part of hemifacial spasm, the patient should undergo magnetic resonance imaging (MRI) to rule out a compressive posterior fossa lesion. If the results are negative, and botulinum injections are ineffective, a suboccipital craniectomy with placement of a sponge between the seventh nerve root and an aberrant vessel is often effective.

WHAT IS THE OUTCOME?

Botulinum toxin injections relieve blepharospasm temporarily in the majority of cases, although serial retreatments (every 2 to 5 months) are usually necessary. Posterior fossa nerve decompression is effective in the majority of patients with hemifacial spasm but carries a small risk of permanent neurologic deficits.

CHAPTER 14
Lid Retraction

WHAT IS IT?

Upward displacement of the upper lid caused by excess innervation or cicatricial shortening of the levator palpebrae superioris. Most cases are due to Graves' disease, an autoimmune inflammation affecting orbital tissues. Other orbital inflammations, trauma, midbrain disease, and hypervigilant states (drug-induced states, psychotic disorders) can also cause it.

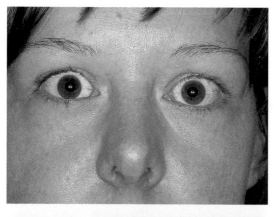

A

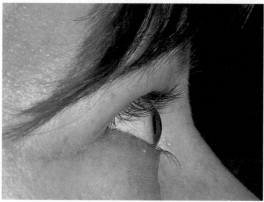

B

FIGURE 1. Lid retraction. **A:** Frontal view shows baring of upper sclera (scleral show). **B:** Side view shows that the scleral show is due to lid retraction, not to forward displacement of the eye (proptosis).

WHAT DOES IT LOOK LIKE?

The upper lid rides too high above the cornea, exposing the superior conjunctiva. In Graves' disease, lid retraction is usually bilateral but may be markedly asymmetric. An associated sign is lid lag: The upper lid initially hangs up during downward rotation of the eye. Lid and conjunctival swelling and hyperemia, proptosis, and eye movement deficits need not be present in Graves' disease.

WHAT ELSE LOOKS LIKE IT?

Proptosis (exophthalmos). However, proptosis must be very severe before the upper conjunctiva becomes exposed. In simple lid retraction, the eye lies in a normal position relative to the orbital margin. When lid retraction is unilateral, be sure that it does not represent an extra effort to raise the eyelids to overcome ptosis in the contralateral eye.

HOW DO YOU DIAGNOSE?

By noting the combination of retraction and lag, and accompanying signs suggesting orbital inflammation (lid and conjunctival swelling, eye movement deficits, proptosis).

HOW DO YOU MANAGE?

Depends on the cause. Unless a diagnosis of Graves' disease is obvious, refer for consultation with a specialist.

WHAT IS THE OUTCOME?

Depends on the cause. In Graves' disease, lid retraction often does not reverse even if hyperthyroidism is relieved. This is because the lid changes have become cicatricial. Under these circumstances, eye exposure can be treated with artificial tears. If this is not sufficient to protect the cornea, the lids can be lowered surgically.

CHAPTER 15

Dacryocystitis

WHAT IS IT?

Infection of the lacrimal sac. This condition is most common in infants who have a blockage of the nasolacrimal drainage system leading from the lid puncta through the lacrimal sac and duct into the nose. In adults, dacryocystitis is the result of chronic sinusitis, facial trauma, or neoplasm.

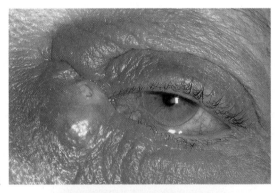

A

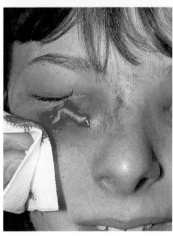

B

FIGURE 1. Dacryocystitis. **A:** Moundlike swelling and redness over the lacrimal sac nasal to the lower lid. **B:** Pus escapes from the lower punctum.

WHAT DOES IT LOOK LIKE?

Tender, erythematous, domelike swelling of the medial lower lid overlying the lacrimal sac. Sometimes mucopurulent discharge emerges from the punctum or a skin fistula, especially following digital pressure on the mass.

WHAT ELSE LOOKS LIKE IT?

Orbital or facial cellulitis, stye. But cellulitis should not be focal. Styes are rarely located so medially on the lid and are never purulent.

HOW DO YOU DIAGNOSE?

By the clinical features. Try to express pus from the punctum for confirmation.

HOW DO YOU MANAGE?

In children under age 1, the presumptive cause is a blocked nasolacrimal duct, and so no additional workup is needed. In those who are older, facial and sinus imaging is indicated. Mild cases respond to topical or oral antibiotics targeted at skin organisms; more severe cases require intravenous antibiotics. If there is no improvement within 24 hours, the lacrimal system must be probed to try to open up any blocking membranes or valves.

WHAT IS THE OUTCOME?

Most cases respond to antibiotics within days. Persistent tearing and recurrent infections suggest a block in the sac or duct and may require lacrimal tubes or surgical diversion (dacryocystorhinostomy).

Orbital Cellulitis

WHAT IS IT?

Bacterial infection of orbital tissues. Most common in children, it originates from an infected ethmoid sinus. Infection usually remains confined to the lids, but it can extend throughout the orbit and into the intracranial space where it becomes life threatening.

Orbital cellulitis is rare in adults. In normal adult hosts, similar signs may be caused by an immunogenic inflammation (Graves' disease, orbital pseudotumor) or a neoplasm. In immunocompromised hosts, particularly diabetic patients, one must fear mucormycosis or aspergillosis, life-threatening illnesses that require prompt management.

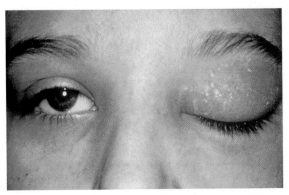

FIGURE 1. Orbital cellulitis. Right eyelids and cheek are diffusely and violaceously swollen.

WHAT DOES IT LOOK LIKE?

Smooth, purplish (violaceous) swelling of both lids usually confined to one side and reaching maximal intensity within a few days. The swelling may be marked enough to cover the eye completely and not allow the lids to be forcefully opened. The conjunctiva may be hyperemic and swollen. In severe cases, the eye has restricted movement. Vision is rarely impaired, however. The patient complains of periocular pain and/or headache. Children often have manifestations of an upper respiratory infection.

In immunocompromised or elderly adults, a slow development of these signs suggests fungal sinoorbital disease caused by mucormycosis or aspergillosis. Both cause a necrotizing vasculitis that kills by thrombosing nutrient vessels. Loss of vision and life is an ever-present concern.

WHAT ELSE LOOKS LIKE IT?

Severe conjunctivitis, dacryocystitis, stye, orbital tumor, noninfectious orbital inflammation, and orbital trauma. In conjunctivitis, the inflammation should be greater in the conjunctiva than in the lids. Dacryocystitis and stye cause focal lid inflammations. Orbital trauma is diagnosed with the appropriate history. Noninfectious orbital inflammation and orbital tumors arise more slowly but may not be excludable without imaging.

HOW DO YOU DIAGNOSE?

But noting acute, nonfocal, violaceous swelling of the eyelids. In most cases, orbital/sinus/brain imaging is necessary for confirmation.

HOW DO YOU MANAGE?

Use imaging to rule out sinusitis, orbital subperiosteal abscess, or a tumor. In children less than 9 years of age, treat for aerobic gram-positive organisms with i.v. ceftriaxone sodium 1 to 2 g t.i.d. for 3 days. In older children and adults, add i.v. clindamycin phosphate 300 mg q.i.d., i.v. vancomycin 1 g b.i.d., or metronidazole 15 mg/kg load and 7.5 mg/kg q.i.d. because of the possibility of anaerobic infection. Lack of improvement within 24 to 48 hours signals either an incorrect diagnosis or ineffective antibacterial agents. A subperiosteal abscess may require surgical drainage. In immunocompromised adults, consider sinus exploration to rule out mucormycosis or other fungi.

WHAT IS THE OUTCOME?

Most cases respond within 24 to 48 hours to i.v. antibiotics. Lack of improvement within this period mandates reimaging and consultation with specialists.

CHAPTER 17
Noninfectious Orbital Inflammation

WHAT IS IT?

Inflammation of the orbital tissues caused by autoimmune conditions including Graves' disease, idiopathic orbital inflammation (orbital pseudotumor), and connective tissue disorders (Wegener's granulomatosis, lupus erythematosus, relapsing polychondritis).

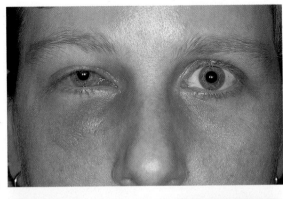

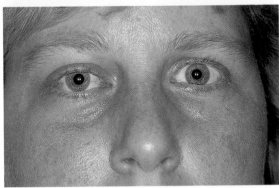

FIGURE 1. Noninfectious orbital inflammation. **A:** Right eyelids and conjunctiva are swollen and hyperemic in a patient with idiopathic orbital inflammation (orbital pseudotumor). **B:** After immunosuppressive treatment, the inflammation is reduced. *(continued)*

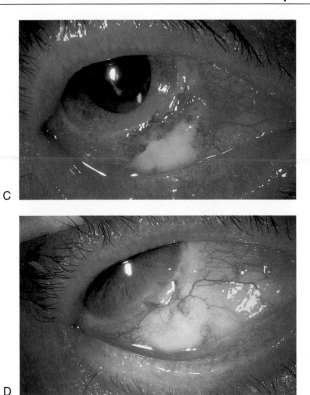

C

D

FIGURE 1. *Continued*. C: Conjunctival hyperemia and scleral necrosis in Wegener's granulomatosis. **D:** After immunosuppressive treatment, the inflammation is reduced and the sclera is healing.

WHAT DOES IT LOOK LIKE?

The patient often complains of periocular pain and tenderness. One or more of the following is found: diffuse lid swelling, diffuse conjunctival hyperemia, proptosis, reduced eye movements, keratitis, scleritis, or uveitis. In Graves' disease, the upper lid is usually retracted and displays lid lag on downward gaze.

WHAT ELSE LOOKS LIKE IT?

Orbital tumor, orbital cellulitis, severe conjunctivitis, carotid-cavernous fistula (CCF). Orbital tumors cause less pain and soft tissue inflammation. Orbital cellulitis is more acute and causes tenser, more violaceous lid swelling. CCFs cause more conjunctival hyperemia, and the patient often reports pulsatile tinnitus. Intraocular pressure is elevated on the affected side, and the retinal veins are often dilated.

Imaging is necessary to differentiate among these entities. Tumors should be obvious as mass lesions; cellulitis is usually accompanied by ethmoid or frontal sinus opacification and perhaps subperiosteal fluid collections; noninfectious inflammation shows swelling of extraocular muscles, lacrimal gland, or sclera, and increased vascular markings in orbital fat. CCFs display a dilated superior ophthalmic vein and sometimes a distended cavernous sinus.

HOW DO YOU DIAGNOSE?

By combining clinical and imaging findings.

HOW DO YOU MANAGE?

Perform orbitocranial imaging to help with the diagnosis. Correct hormonal abnormalities in Graves' disease but remember that the congestive orbital soft tissue manifestations are not affected by this treatment. When vision is depressed by compression of the optic nerve, begin high-dose corticosteroids promptly, followed by surgical decompression of the orbit by removal of its medial and inferior walls. Local radiation is an alternative treatment for Graves' optic neuropathy.

The congestive orbital manifestations may be partially relieved with sympathomimetic eyedrops, systemic diuretics, and head-of-bed elevation. The use of short courses of oral corticosteroids is controversial. These agents provide only brief benefit; chronic use brings on toxicity.

In suspected orbital pseudotumor, the patient should be screened for associated autoimmune diseases. If the results are negative, treat with a 14-day course of oral prednisone (1 mg/kg/day). If the manifestations keep recurring on corticosteroid withdrawal, reimage the patient and consider biopsy of an orbital mass. If no mass is present, treat with low-dose (1,500 to 2,000 Gy) orbital x-irradiation.

WHAT IS THE OUTCOME?

Depends on the cause. In mild Graves' ophthalmopathy, the soft tissue signs regress spontaneously within 2 years. More severe cases usually cause permanent lid retraction from scarring of the levator palpebrae superioris and diplopia from scarring of extraocular muscles. Surgical correction is often effective in restoring normal lid position and ocular alignment, but several procedures may be necessary.

Orbital pseudotumor is usually effectively treated by oral corticosteroids or x-irradiation but may recur. Orbital inflammation in connective tissue disease typically requires systemic medication directed at the underlying illness.

Orbital Tumor

WHAT IS IT?

A mass lesion of the orbit. It may be solid or cystic, cellular or vascular, benign or malignant, primary or metastatic.

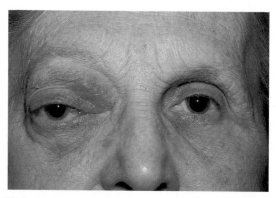

FIGURE 1. Orbital tumor. The right eye is proptotic, and its eyelids are swollen and congested.

WHAT DOES IT LOOK LIKE?

Most orbital tumors cause slowly progressive displacement of the eye, usually forward (proptosis, exophthalmos) but sometimes upward or downward. Patients usually experience some discomfort or a sensation of fullness around the eye, but they rarely have much pain. The notable exceptions to this indolent presentation are metastatic tumors, lymphomas, and varices. If eye movement is restricted, the patient will report diplopia. Vision is often preserved.

WHAT ELSE LOOKS LIKE IT?

Noninfectious orbital inflammation and carotid-cavernous fistula (CCF). But both cause more inflammatory signs and develop more rapidly.

HOW DO YOU DIAGNOSE?

By clinical, imaging, and histologic findings. Superficial tumors can be biopsied; deep tumors are hard to reach without causing damage to sight. In these deep tumors, try to make a diagnosis indirectly by finding a primary tumor elsewhere.

HOW DO YOU MANAGE?

Depends on the type of tumor. Observation, surgical extirpation, radiation, and systemic chemotherapy are considerations.

WHAT IS THE OUTCOME?

Depends on the type of tumor.

CHAPTER 19
Carotid-Cavernous Fistula

WHAT IS IT?

An abnormal communication between the carotid artery or its branches and the veins of the cavernous sinus. This shunt can be created by head trauma or occur spontaneously. Under high pressure, blood is forced retrograde into the ophthalmic veins, creating a congestive orbitopathy. Postpartum and postmenopausal women are at particular risk for spontaneous fistulas.

WHAT DOES IT LOOK LIKE?

Patients report discomfort around the affected orbit, and sometimes diplopia and pulsatile tinnitus. Vision may be impaired. Examination discloses swollen lids, proptosis, reduced eye movements, elevated intraocular pressure, dilated retinal veins, and a characteristic "corkscrew" distention and tortuosity of conjunctival veins.

WHAT ELSE LOOKS LIKE IT?

Noninfectious orbital inflammation and orbital tumor. But both cause more inflammatory signs and develop more rapidly.

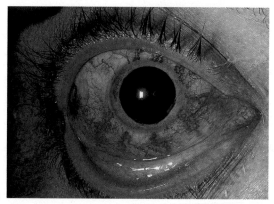

A

FIGURE 1. Carotid-cavernous fistula (CCF). **A:** "Corkscrew" distention and tortuosity of conjunctival veins. *(continued)*

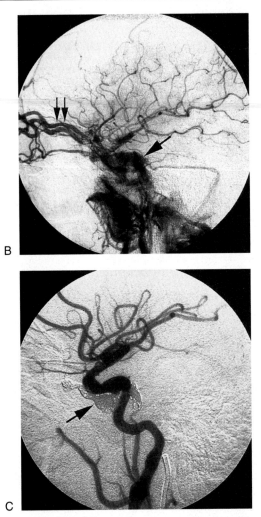

FIGURE 1. *Continued*. B: Arteriogram showing fistula (*single arrow*) and dilated orbital veins (*double arrows*). **C:** After endovascular closure of fistula with coils implanted in the cavernous sinus *(arrow)*, orbital veins are no longer dilated.

HOW DO YOU DIAGNOSE?

By clinical and imaging findings. Computed tomography (CT) and magnetic resonance imaging (MRI) often show a dilated superior ophthalmic vein in the orbit. Catheter cerebral angiography, the only way to make a definitive diagnosis, reveals an arteriovenous shunt in the region of the cavernous sinus.

HOW DO YOU MANAGE?

Traumatic and high-flow fistulas must be closed by embolizing coils into the fistula through the carotid arteries or petrosal veins. Performed by interventional radiologists, these procedures require great expertise. Low-flow (dural) fistulas often close spontaneously within months; they can be left alone unless the patient has intolerable pain, very high intraocular pressure, or visual loss.

WHAT IS THE OUTCOME?

Embolic closure of fistulas is often successful, but stroke is a risk. Dural fistulas that have multiple feeders may be difficult to close, even with expert technique.

CHAPTER 20

Lid Laceration

WHAT IS IT?

A traumatic cut through the lid. It may be simple or complex. Complex lacerations are those that cut through the lid margin, the lower canaliculus, or the medial canthal tendon, or cause large areas of avulsed tissue or prolapsed orbital fat. Their repair requires special expertise.

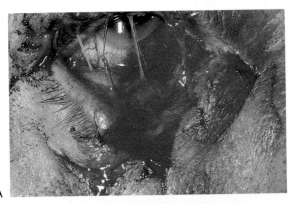

A

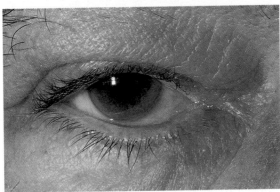

B

FIGURE 1. Lid laceration. **A:** Lower lid is torn at its margin in a complex laceration. **B:** Months after skilled suturing, the lid has healed with a smooth margin that is properly apposed to the eye.

WHAT DOES IT LOOK LIKE?

Most lid lacerations are easy to recognize unless the tissue is swollen and badly distorted.

WHAT ELSE LOOKS LIKE IT?

Nothing.

HOW DO YOU DIAGNOSE?

By observation. In complex cases, the relationship of the laceration to the canaliculus and its full extent are discovered by anesthetizing the patient and using special instruments.

HOW DO YOU MANAGE?

Simple lacerations can be closed by interrupted 6-0 absorbable or non-absorbable sutures. Complex lacerations should be handled by a specialist.

WHAT IS THE OUTCOME?

Simple lid lacerations are usually easy to suture and resolve without cosmetic defect. The outcome of repaired complex lacerations depends on their location and on the expertise of the operator.

CHAPTER 21

Orbital Wall Fracture

WHAT IS IT?

A fracture through one or more of the walls of the orbit. The most common areas involved are the orbital floor and lamina papyracea of the ethmoid sinus on the medial orbital wall. Such fractures are caused by displacement of the globe or by direct impact on the orbital rim. Fracture of the orbital rim itself signifies a severe blow. Superior rim fractures are a particular concern because of possible associated fractures through the frontal sinus and calvarium.

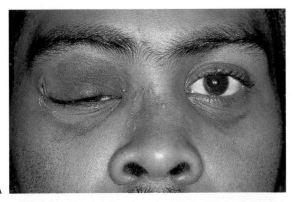

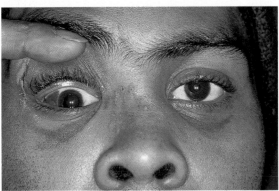

FIGURE 1. Orbital wall fracture. **A:** Deep hemorrhage within right lids suggests severe soft tissue contusion. **B:** Right eye is lower than left because the right inferior rectus is trapped within an orbital floor fracture.

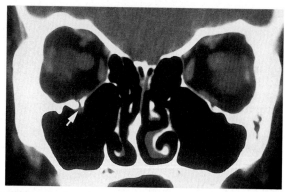

FIGURE 1. *Continued.* C: Orbital floor fracture is visible on a computed tomography (CT) scan as a discontinuity in bone *(arrow).*

WHAT DOES IT LOOK LIKE?

Most patients have considerable lid swelling and sometimes lacerations, often with conjunctival hemorrhage. The eye itself may be contused or lacerated. A large intraorbital hemorrhage may cause proptosis and markedly elevated intraocular pressure.

Inferior wall fractures may cause entrapment of the inferior rectus muscle and prevent full upward or downward movement of the eye. Medial wall fractures may prevent full inward or outward movement. Rim fractures can sometimes be palpated as discontinuities.

Orbital fractures are diagnosed on computed tomography (CT) imaging as gaps or displacements of bone; air may be visible in the orbit, and a fluid level is often seen in the maxillary sinus.

WHAT ELSE LOOKS LIKE IT?

Nothing; a history of trauma makes the diagnosis.

HOW DO YOU DIAGNOSE?

By imaging.

HOW DO YOU MANAGE?

Be sure that the eye is unharmed. Suspect trouble if visual acuity is impaired. Inspect for blood in the anterior chamber (hyphema), an irregular, poorly reactive pupil, or lack of a red reflex. If the conjunctiva is hemorrhagic, suspect a retrobulbar hemorrhage, which might be raising the intraocular pressure to dangerously high levels. If so, emergency surgical release of the lateral canthal tendon (canthotomy and catholysis) is necessary to allow the eye room to move forward.

Rim fractures are usually repaired within days if sufficiently displaced. Orbital wall fractures do not require emergent repair. Orbital floor fractures are repaired 7 to 14 days later with the insertion of a plate if the eye is sunken inward and downward or does not move vertically. Some physicians prescribe an oral cephalosporin or erythromycin to prevent orbital infection from the spread of sinus organisms. If the eye is contused, ophthalmologic evaluation is necessary.

WHAT IS THE OUTCOME?

Most orbital fractures do not cause long-term problems of ocular motility unless they are severe. Postponing surgical repair of floor fractures is prudent because it allows the soft tissue swelling to resolve and reveal whether eye position and motility are normal.

CHAPTER 22

Third Cranial Nerve Palsy

WHAT IS IT?

A lesion of the third cranial nerve, usually in its course outside the brainstem. Although head trauma, meningeal lesions, and ischemia are the principal causes, a major concern is a compressive mass such as a cerebral aneurysm.

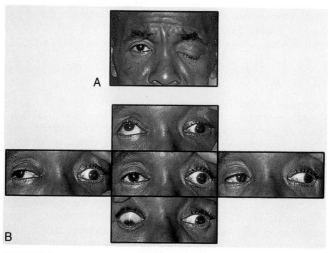

FIGURE 1. Left third cranial nerve palsy. **A:** Left upper lid ptosis. **B:** Abducted left eye **(center)**, absent left adduction **(left)**, full left abduction **(right)**, absent left supraduction **(top)**, and absent left infraduction **(bottom)**.

WHAT DOES IT LOOK LIKE?

The patient complains of diplopia and a droopy upper lid. A severe lesion causes ipsilateral complete ptosis, paralysis of adduction, supraduction, and infraduction, and a dilated (mydriatic) pupil that does not constrict to direct light. Subtotal lesions may damage all these functions to a lesser degree or spare some of them entirely. A fixed, dilated pupil suggests a compressive lesion, including an aneurysm; a normal pupil does not exclude it.

WHAT ELSE LOOKS LIKE IT?

One or more of the findings can be caused by myasthenia gravis, a medial longitudinal fasciculus (MLF) lesion, or an orbital lesion. But myasthenia gravis never affects the pupil. MLF lesions cause only slowed or limited adduction. Orbital lesions can usually be distinguished by the presence of proptosis, soft tissue swelling, or resistance to retropulsing the eye.

HOW DO YOU DIAGNOSE?

By the characteristic clinical manifestations. Mild lesions are hard to diagnose because they cause partial palsies. Isolated ptosis or isolated mydriasis is virtually never caused by a third cranial nerve palsy.

HOW DO YOU MANAGE?

Because of the threat of aneurysm, refer promptly to an ophthalmologist, neuro-ophthalmologist, or neurologist. The workup usually includes emergent magnetic resonance imaging (MRI), magnetic resonance angiography (MRA), and possibly catheter cerebral angiography.

WHAT IS THE OUTCOME?

Depends on the cause. Ischemic lesions usually resolve spontaneously within 3 months. Aneurysmal repair may lead to full recovery. Traumatic damage often leaves a permanent deficit, although mild damage may resolve. For persistent palsies, eye muscle surgery may restore satisfactory ocular alignment if the preoperative deficits are mild.

CHAPTER 23

Fourth Cranial Nerve Palsy

WHAT IS IT?

A lesion of the fourth cranial nerve, usually in its course outside the brainstem. As with third cranial nerve palsy, head trauma, meningeal lesions, and ischemia are common causes. A congenital lesion, held in check until adulthood, may become apparent for unclear reasons. Compressive lesions, including aneurysm, are rarely responsible.

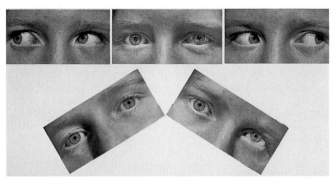

FIGURE 1. Left fourth cranial nerve palsy. Left eye is higher in straight-ahead gaze (**center**), right gaze (**left**), and left head tilt (**lower right**); eyes are aligned in left gaze (**right**) and right head tilt (**lower left**).

WHAT DOES IT LOOK LIKE?

The patient complains of diplopia, one image above the other. One image often appears tilted. Severe lesions cause reduced infraduction in adduction on the affected side, but this is usually difficult to detect. The images are farthest apart with gaze away from the side of the lesion and with head tilt in the direction of the lesion.

WHAT ELSE LOOKS LIKE IT?

Vertical diplopia may be caused by a brainstem lesion (skew deviation), myasthenia gravis, an orbital lesion, or a third cranial nerve palsy. Brainstem lesions usually cause other neurologic manifestations (nystagmus, ataxia); myasthenia gravis often causes ptosis; orbital lesions often produce proptosis, swelling of soft tissues, and resistance to retropulsion of the eye.

HOW DO YOU DIAGNOSE?

By finding vertical diplopia that worsens on gaze contralateral and on head tilt ipsilateral to the side of the lesion. Even with these findings, other causes cannot be entirely excluded.

HOW DO YOU MANAGE?

Diagnosis is hard enough to merit evaluation by an ophthalmologist, neuro-ophthalmologist, or neurologist. Brain imaging is often unnecessary.

WHAT IS THE OUTCOME?

Depends on the cause. Ischemic lesions usually resolve spontaneously within 3 months. Traumatic damage often leaves a permanent deficit, although mild damage may resolve. Decompensated congenital palsies usually do not resolve. For persistent palsies, eye muscle surgery is often successful in restoring ocular alignment.

CHAPTER 24
Sixth Cranial Nerve Palsy

WHAT IS IT?

A lesion of the sixth cranial nerve, usually in its course outside the brainstem. As with third and fourth cranial nerve palsies, common causes are head trauma, meningeal lesions, and ischemia. In addition, increased and decreased intracranial pressure may also produce sixth cranial nerve palsy. Compressive lesions are also frequently responsible, but not aneurysms.

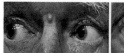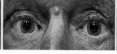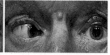

FIGURE 1. Left sixth cranial nerve palsy. Esotropia (convergent misalignment) is present in straight-ahead gaze (**center**); eyes are aligned in right gaze (**left**); the misalignment worsens in left gaze because the left eye does not abduct (**right**).

WHAT DOES IT LOOK LIKE?

The patient complains of horizontal diplopia. Severe lesions cause complete loss of abduction on the affected side. Lesser lesions produce partial abduction deficits. The eyes are convergently misaligned, with image separation greatest in gaze toward the side of the lesion.

WHAT ELSE LOOKS LIKE IT?

Myasthenia gravis, an orbital lesion, and excessive convergence (caused by a variety of intracranial lesions or by malingering or anxiety).

HOW DO YOU DIAGNOSE?

By finding either an abduction deficit or a convergent misalignment in the presence of diplopia.

HOW DO YOU MANAGE?

Diagnosis is hard enough to merit evaluation by an ophthalmologist, neuro-ophthalmologist, or neurologist. Brain imaging is usually necessary.

WHAT IS THE OUTCOME?

Depends on the cause. Ischemic lesions usually resolve spontaneously within 3 months. Traumatic damage often leaves a permanent deficit, although mild damage may resolve. For persistent palsies, eye muscle surgery is often successful in restoring ocular alignment.

CHAPTER 25

Viral Conjunctivitis

WHAT IS IT?

An infection of the conjunctiva caused by a variety of viruses, many of which are very contagious. It accounts for more than 95% of cases of unilateral acute red eye. Often part of an adenovirus upper respiratory infection, it is unpleasant but short-lived and not vision threatening.

WHAT DOES IT LOOK LIKE?

The patient complains of a tight, warm, sometimes scratchy feeling in the affected eye. The lids are swollen, the conjunctiva is diffusely hy-

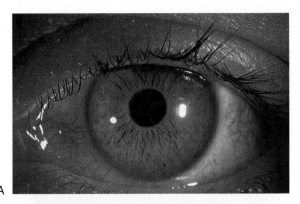
A

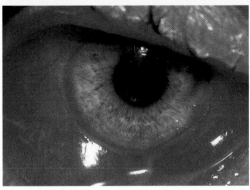
B

FIGURE 1. Viral conjunctivitis. **A:** Conjunctiva is mildly and diffusely hyperemic. **B:** Conjunctiva is bullous (chemosis) and fiery red.

peremic, and the discharge is watery. Only one eye is affected—at least initially. The preauricular node on the affected side is enlarged and tender. The cornea is usually normal. Vision should be unaffected.

WHAT ELSE LOOKS LIKE IT?

Allergic conjunctivitis, keratitis, uveitis, and acute angle closure glaucoma. Allergic conjunctivitis is always bilateral and usually itchy. In keratitis, the cornea stains with fluorescein dye or displays an opacity; the patient often complains of photophobia and a foreign body sensation. In uveitis, the pupil is often irregular; the patient reports photophobia and aching periocular or brow pain. In acute angle closure glaucoma, the cornea is often cloudy, intraocular pressure is markedly elevated, and vision is reduced; the patient complains of blurred vision and severe periocular pain.

HOW DO YOU DIAGNOSE?

By finding diffuse conjunctival hyperemia, a watery discharge, a tender, swollen preauricular node, normal vision, and a normal cornea.

HOW DO YOU MANAGE?

Do not treat. Antiinfectives are useless. Instilling artificial tears or sterile ointments does not reduce discomfort; it merely increases the chances of spreading the infection to the other eye and to other individuals. Tell patients to avoid touching their eyes, to wash their hands frequently, and to use separate towels and utensils. As long as there is a discharge, the condition is contagious. Patients ideally should avoid communal activities (work, school, and daycare) for that period. Refer immunocompetent patients only if there is initial doubt about the diagnosis, if symptoms and signs persist beyond a week, or if manifestations evolve into an atypical complex.

WHAT IS THE OUTCOME?

It resolves spontaneously without sequelae within a week. Rarely, the cornea may become involved.

CHAPTER 26
Bacterial Conjunctivitis

WHAT IS IT?

Infection of the conjunctiva by a bacterium. Extraordinarily rare in the ordinary host, it arises primarily among the immunocompromised, neonates, contact lens wearers, and those who suffer ocular surface trauma. The common pathogens are *Staphylococcus aureus*, *Streptococcus pneumoniae*, and *Haemophilus influenzae*. *Pseudomonas* organisms, *Neisseria gonorrhoeae*, and anaerobes are the most dangerous organisms, producing a rapid necrosis that is hard to stop even with appropriate topical and systemic treatment.

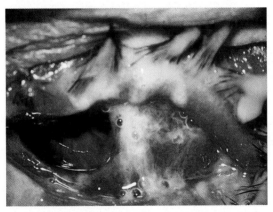

FIGURE 1. Bacterial conjunctivitis. Eyelids and conjunctiva are swollen, red, and purulent.

WHAT DOES IT LOOK LIKE?

The patient complains of marked discomfort. The lids are very swollen, the conjunctiva is both swollen (chemotic) and hyperemic, and the discharge is purulent.

WHAT ELSE LOOKS LIKE IT?

Severe viral and allergic conjunctivitis, carotid-cavernous fistula (CCF), and orbital cellulitis. Viral conjunctivitis and allergic conjunctivitis have a mucoid discharge; viral conjunctivitis usually has an inflamed preauricular node; allergic conjunctivitis is usually bilateral and itches; CCF and orbital cellulitis do not cause purulence.

HOW DO YOU DIAGNOSE?

By finding swollen lids, fiery-red and swollen conjunctivae, and purulence.

HOW DO YOU MANAGE?

For mild bacterial conjunctivitis, use topical sulfa, tobramycin, ciprofloxacin, or norfloxacin. For suspected *Neisseria*, *Pseudomonas*, or anaerobic conjunctivitis, treatment involves fortified topical, periocular, and systemic agents and is best left to an ophthalmologist.

Quarantine is not necessary because of the low degree of contagiousness. Refer all immunocompromised hosts, neonates, contact lens wearers, those with ocular trauma, and those with worsening signs after 3 days of treatment or lack of improvement after 7 days.

WHAT IS THE OUTCOME?

Depends on the host, the organism, and the timeliness and intensity of treatment. *Neisseria*, *Pseudomonas*, and anaerobes may cause blinding keratitis or endophthalmitis.

CHAPTER 27
Allergic Conjunctivitis

WHAT IS IT?

A hyperimmune reaction of the conjunctiva to exogenous or endogenous allergens. Other mucous membranes usually participate—especially the nose and throat. Except for the rare serious variants (Stevens-Johnson syndrome, graft-vs-host disease), it is not vision threatening, but it causes a lot of misery.

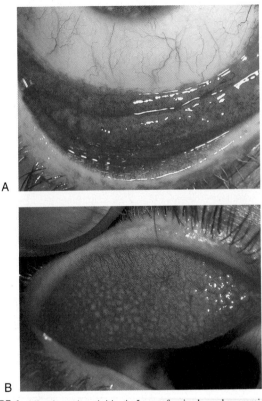

FIGURE 1. Allergic conjunctivitis. **A:** Lower fornix shows hyperemic, swollen mucosa. **B:** Mucosa of upper lid shows papillary hypertrophy.

WHAT DOES IT LOOK LIKE?

Lid swelling and bilateral, boggy, hyperemic conjunctiva with stringy mucoid discharge. The eyes itch. Rubbing them only makes the inflammation worse.

WHAT ELSE LOOKS LIKE IT?

Other conditions that produce chronically red eyes, including blepharitis, chlamydial conjunctivitis, and keratitis sicca (dry eye syndrome). Blepharitis causes a gritty rather than an itchy sensation; the lid margins are crusty. Chlamydial conjunctivitis is often unilateral and does not cause itching or boggy swelling of the lids or conjunctiva. Keratitis sicca causes a foreign body sensation and photophobia; the cornea usually stains with fluorescein.

HOW DO YOU DIAGNOSE?

By finding the combination of watery discharge, boggy/hyperemic conjunctiva, and itchiness in a patient with other symptoms of mucosal allergy.

HOW DO YOU MANAGE?

Try oral antiallergic medications first. If they do not work, prescribe topical vasoconstrictor/antihistamine combinations (naphazoline/pheniramine and others). If that is no help, move on to topical H-1 blockers (levocabastine, emedastine, olopatadine), mast cell stabilizers (cromolyn, lodoxamide), or ketorolac. Topical steroids should generally be avoided because of their ocular and systemic side effects.

WHAT IS THE OUTCOME?

Symptoms are usually adequately palliated with a combination of oral and topical agents.

Chlamydial Conjunctivitis

WHAT IS IT?

A chronic conjunctivitis caused by *Chlamydia trachomatis* that occurs in two forms: (a) neonatal, acquired from an infected cervix, and (b) adult, acquired by sexual contact. The neonatal form is the commonest cause of a red eye in a newborn. The adult form is an indolent conjunctivitis resistant to standard topical antibiotics. It is often accompanied by vaginitis, cervicitis, or urethritis that is often asymptomatic. Diagnosis is frequently delayed.

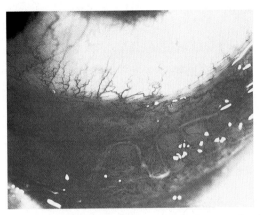

FIGURE 1. Chlamydial conjunctivitis. Fornix shows bumpy red conjunctiva full of lymphoid follicles outlined by stringy mucus.

WHAT DOES IT LOOK LIKE?

In neonates, mild to severe conjunctival hyperemia with a mucoid discharge. In adults, a mild chronic conjunctival hyperemia with prominent follicles on the inferior tarsal and bulbar conjunctivae. The ipsilateral preauricular node is usually enlarged but not very tender. The condition may be monocular or binocular.

WHAT ELSE LOOKS LIKE IT?

In neonates, the differential diagnosis includes conjunctivitis caused by antiseptic chemical instillation, bacteria (*Neisseria*, *Streptococcus*, *Staphylococcus*, *Haemophilus*, gram-negative organisms), and herpes simplex Type 2. In adults, it is mimicked by allergic conjunctivitis, ble-pharitis, and keratitis sicca (dry eye syndrome). But allergic conjunc-tivitis is seasonal and causes boggy rather than follicular inflammation. Blepharitis causes a gritty sensation, and the lid margins are crusty. Keratitis sicca causes a foreign body sensation and photophobia; the cornea usually stains with fluorescein.

HOW DO YOU DIAGNOSE?

First, by suspecting the diagnosis in a neonate with a red eye and in an adult with a chronic red eye unresponsive to antibiotic drops. Second, by finding basophilic intracytoplasmic inclusions and a positive direct fluorescent antibody stain of conjunctival scrapings.

HOW DO YOU MANAGE?

Treat neonates with topical tetracycline ointment four times daily and oral erythromycin for 4 weeks. Treat parents with oral doxycycline or erythromycin for 4 weeks. Treat adults and their sexual partners with oral doxycycline or erythromycin.

WHAT IS THE OUTCOME?

Treatment is usually effective in eradicating the disease and leaving no sequelae.

CHAPTER 29

Erythema Multiforme Major Conjunctivitis (Stevens-Johnson Syndrome)

WHAT IS IT?

An allergic reaction of skin and mucous membranes usually attributed to systemic ingestion of a medication such as a sulfonamide, penicillin, phenytoin, barbiturate, tetracycline, thiazide, or phenylbutazone. In 50% of cases, there is a raging conjunctivitis.

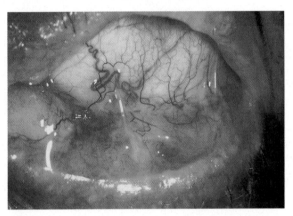

FIGURE 1. Stevens-Johnson syndrome. Chronic phase: Palpebral and bulbar conjunctivae are scarred to one another, shortening the fornix and eliminating tear-producing glands.

WHAT DOES IT LOOK LIKE?

The lids are swollen, and the conjunctiva is raised in bullae (chemosis) with dramatic vessel engorgement and hemorrhage. The inflammation typically evolves over several days and may lead to cicatricial adhesion of the tarsal and bulbar conjunctivae (symblepharon). The cornea is spared. The condition always affects both eyes, but sometimes asymmetrically.

WHAT ELSE LOOKS LIKE IT?

An insect bite of the conjunctiva may cause the same reaction but is always unilateral. Severe viral conjunctivitis resembles it but usually has a swollen preauricular node. Bacterial conjunctivitis is more purulent.

HOW DO YOU DIAGNOSE?

By noting the accompanying skin and mucous membrane lesions. The skin lesions are red-centered vesicles surrounded by a pale ring (target lesions) and are concentrated on palms and soles. The mucous membrane lesions are crusty bullae of the mouth and urogenital regions.

HOW DO YOU MANAGE?

Eliminate the putative offending agent. Systemic corticosteroids are generally administered, although their benefit is not proven. There is no known effective treatment for the conjunctivitis. Conventional approaches include topical corticosteroids, artificial tears, and ointment. There are advocates of intermittent sweeping of the fornices with a glass rod to prevent symblepharon formation.

WHAT IS THE OUTCOME?

Mild cases resolve without sequelae. Severe cases cause trichiasis (turning in of lashes toward the cornea) and symblepharon, with destruction of the tear-producing tissues, leading to corneal desiccation and blindness. Conjunctival stem cell grafts are showing promise in restoring vision in severe cases.

CHAPTER 30

Chronic Immunogenic Conjunctivitis

WHAT IS IT?

Low-grade sterile conjunctival inflammation associated with chronic immune-mediated diseases such as Graves' disease, lupus erythematosus, rheumatoid arthritis, scleroderma, Sjögren's syndrome, polychondritis, Behçet's disease, and the vasculitic syndromes.

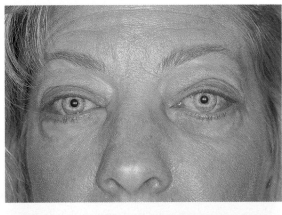

A

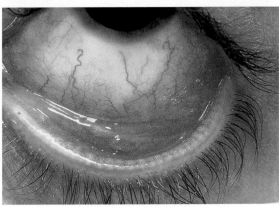

B

FIGURE 1. Chronic immunogenic conjunctivitis. **A:** Graves' disease. The conjunctiva is hyperemic and slightly swollen. **B:** Behçet's disease. The fornical conjunctiva is hyperemic. These signs are nonspecific.

WHAT DOES IT LOOK LIKE?

The conjunctiva is mildly and diffusely hyperemic. If there is any discharge, it is scant. The patient may have no ophthalmic complaints except that the eyes look red and feel slightly irritated.

WHAT ELSE LOOKS LIKE IT?

Ocular cicatricial pemphigoid, dry eye syndrome, and chlamydial, chemical, and factitious conjunctivitis. Pemphigoid usually produces symblepharon; chemical conjunctivitis is diagnosed by a history of topical medication or lid cosmetic exposure. Chlamydial conjunctivitis has follicles. Factitious conjunctivitis, or conjunctivitis self-induced by repeated rubbing of the eyes or insertion of foreign bodies, may be hard to distinguish.

HOW DO YOU DIAGNOSE?

By linking the eye findings to other rheumatologic manifestations. (In many patients, this link goes unnoticed for long periods during which their conjunctivitis is treated unsuccessfully with topical antibiotics.)

HOW DO YOU MANAGE?

By treating the underlying systemic condition.

WHAT IS THE OUTCOME?

Resolution depends on the success in overcoming the systemic condition.

CHAPTER 31
Chemical Conjunctivitis

WHAT IS IT?

Conjunctivitis caused by topical ocular medications, lid cosmetics, or environmental pollutants.

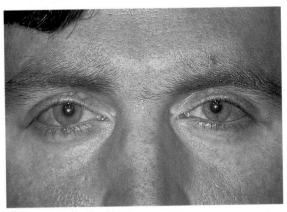

FIGURE 1. Chemical conjunctivitis. Conjunctiva is diffusely hyperemic in both eyes from chemical irritation.

WHAT DOES IT LOOK LIKE?

The patient complains of mild irritation or photophobia. The conjunctiva is mildly and diffusely hyperemic with scant discharge.

WHAT ELSE LOOKS LIKE IT?

Ocular cicatricial pemphigoid, dry eye syndrome, chlamydial conjunctivitis, chemical conjunctivitis, and factitious conjunctivitis. Pemphigoid usually produces symblepharon; chlamydial conjunctivitis has follicles. Factitious conjunctivitis, or conjunctivitis self-induced by repeated rubbing of the eyes or insertion of foreign bodies, may be hard to distinguish.

HOW DO YOU DIAGNOSE?

By linking the eye manifestations in time to exposure to potential toxic irritants, eliminating them if possible, and observing recovery.

HOW DO YOU MANAGE?

By eliminating exposure to the offending agents if possible.

WHAT IS THE OUTCOME?

Resolution usually occurs within days to weeks of removing exposure to the responsible agent.

CHAPTER 32
Herpes Simplex Keratitis

WHAT IS IT?

Inflammation of the cornea by herpes simplex virus Type 1.

WHAT DOES IT LOOK LIKE?

The patient complains of a foreign body sensation, photophobia, and sometimes blurred vision. Fluorescein stains areas of devitalized ep-

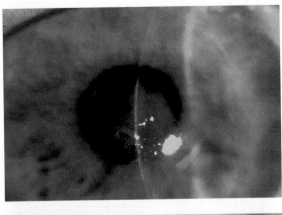

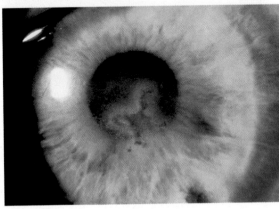

FIGURE 1. Herpes simplex keratitis. **A:** Subtle gray central corneal opacity. **B:** Topical fluorescein outlines a four-pronged epithelial defect. *(continued)*

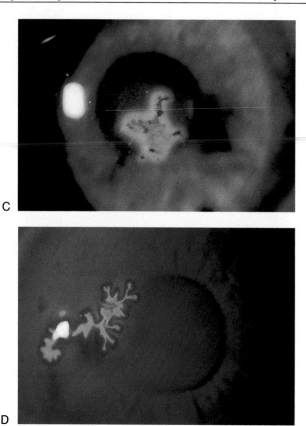

FIGURE 1. *Continued.* C: Cobalt-blue light highlights the defect.
D: Fluorescein highlights a typical dendritic herpes simplex epithelial
lesion in another patient.

ithelium a bright-green color best seen under cobalt-blue light. The
conjunctiva is usually hyperemic, especially near the cornea (ciliary
flush, circumcorneal injection).

WHAT ELSE LOOKS LIKE IT?

Corneal abrasion—traumatic erosion of the epithelium—produces a
patch of fluorescein staining.

HOW DO YOU DIAGNOSE?

By examining the cornea with a bright light, preferably with instruments that allow a magnified view (slit lamp biomicroscope, loupe), and by instilling fluorescein dye and observing with a cobalt-blue light filter (available on newer model direct ophthalmoscopes).

HOW DO YOU MANAGE?

With topical trifluridine or vidarabine or with oral acyclovir. Because improperly managed keratitis can lead to blindness, management should be carried out by specialists.

WHAT IS THE OUTCOME?

Depends on the extent and chronicity of the lesions. Most cases resolve without scarring the cornea, but recurrences are common, possibly triggered by illness, fatigue, stress, and intense sunlight exposure. In severely scarred or thinned corneas, corneal transplantation is the only way to restore vision.

CHAPTER 33
Dry Eye Syndrome

WHAT IS IT?

Damage to the corneal epithelium from inadequate production of tears. Common causes are connective tissue diseases, tumors, ocular radiation, drugs, and cicatricial conjunctival diseases. In pregnant, middle-aged, and elderly women, dry eye syndrome may be an isolated condition.

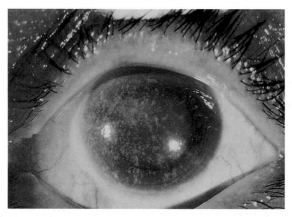

FIGURE 1. Dry eye syndrome. Fluorescein stains multiple punctate epithelial defects.

WHAT DOES IT LOOK LIKE?

The patient complains of a foreign body sensation, photophobia, and sometimes blurred vision. Fluorescein stains tiny punctate areas of devitalized epithelium a bright-green color best seen under cobalt-blue light. Slit lamp biomicroscopy shows early breakup of the tear film after blinking and a reduced tear meniscus on the lower lid margin. The conjunctiva may be hyperemic.

WHAT ELSE LOOKS LIKE IT?

Exposure keratitis from poor lid apposition (seventh nerve palsy, senile ectropion), herpes simplex keratitis, contact lens overwear syndrome, entropion with turned-in eyelashes, and corneal abrasion. However, exposure keratitis typically causes fluorescein staining of the inferior third of the cornea; herpes simplex causes one or more dendritic patches of stain; turned-in lashes (trichiasis) should be evident with slit lamp biomicroscopy; and corneal abrasion usually produces a single round or linear area of staining.

HOW DO YOU DIAGNOSE?

By examining the cornea with a bright light, and preferably with instruments that allow a magnified view (slit lamp biomicroscope, loupe), and by instilling fluorescein dye and observing with a cobalt-blue light filter (available on newer model direct ophthalmoscopes). Reduced tear production is confirmed by the Schirmer test, in which the eyes are topically anesthetized and standard filter paper is placed on the lower lateral palpebral margins. The amount of wetting is measured at 5 minutes; less than 10 mm suggests a tear deficiency.

HOW DO YOU MANAGE?

Mild cases respond to any type of artificial tear instillation. The patient should instill tears as often as is convenient to prevent discomfort. Moderate cases require more viscous tear preparations, which come in single-dose, preservative-free dispensers (Refresh Plus, Celluvisc). Bedtime instillation of a sterile ointment is useful (Refresh PM, Lacri-Lube). Severe cases may also require occlusion of the lacrimal puncta by collagen or silicone inserts (temporary) or by thermal cautery (permanent).

WHAT IS THE OUTCOME?

Depends on how dry the eyes are. All but the most severe cases respond to the suggested measures, which are in the domain of ophthalmologists.

CHAPTER 34
Corneal Abrasion

WHAT IS IT?

Traumatic erosion of the corneal epithelium. Common causes are branches, fingernails, contact lenses, and airborne foreign bodies.

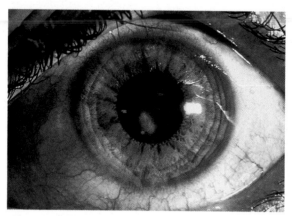

FIGURE 1. Corneal abrasion. Linear green stain in the central cornea.

WHAT DOES IT LOOK LIKE?

The patient complains of a foreign body sensation, photophobia, and sometimes blurred vision. Fluorescein staining usually reveals a linear or round patch of bright-green denuded epithelium best seen under cobalt-blue light. A fuzzy white patch around the erosion suggests an infection.

WHAT ELSE LOOKS LIKE IT?

Dry eye syndrome, infectious or exposure keratitis, and erosion of poorly healed epithelium from prior corneal trauma. The history of recent trauma is a critical feature in differential diagnosis.

HOW DO YOU DIAGNOSE?

By linking the history to the corneal findings.

HOW DO YOU MANAGE?

Topically anesthetize the affected eye and measure visual acuity. Confirm the abrasion with fluorescein staining and make sure there is no corneal laceration. If there is a history of an airborne foreign body, it might be lodged under the upper lid. Look for it by everting the upper lid and inspecting the tarsal sulcus; remove any foreign body with a wet applicator.

Treating with topical antibiotics and cycloplegics is optional. If you choose to do so, use erythromycin ointment for 1 day. Instillation of a topical cycloplegic agent (cyclopentolate 1%, 1 drop) to reduce the pain of ciliary spasm is advisable if the abrasion covers more than one-fourth of the corneal area.

Pressure patching is controversial. For abrasions not caused by contact lenses or vegetable matter, it is safe and induces comfort. Otherwise do not use it because it reduces the antiseptic powers of normal tear flow.

Patients should return for a follow-up examination within 48 hours to make sure the epithelium is healing and that infection has not supervened.

WHAT IS THE OUTCOME?

Most corneal abrasions resolve without scarring within 48 hours. But large, deep scratches may take much longer to heal, can lead to recurrent erosions, and rarely become infected.

CHAPTER 35

Corneal Foreign Body

WHAT IS IT?

Particulate material, usually airborne, that becomes embedded in the superficial cornea. Particles traveling at high velocity can penetrate deeply and even perforate the cornea.

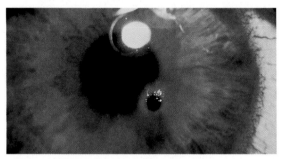

FIGURE 1. Corneal foreign body. Brown spot at the pupil margin.

WHAT DOES IT LOOK LIKE?

The patient complains of a foreign body sensation, photophobia, and sometimes blurred vision. Direct inspection often shows a dark spot on the cornea. If the foreign body is metallic and has been in the cornea for more than 24 hours, it may have spawned a 1-mm rust ring.

WHAT ELSE LOOKS LIKE IT?

Nothing.

HOW DO YOU DIAGNOSE?

By linking the symptoms and the corneal findings.

HOW DO YOU MANAGE?

Topically anesthetize the affected eye and measure visual acuity. Inspect the cornea to rule out a perforation and stain with fluorescein to rule out abrasions. Attempt removal of a superficial foreign body with a wet applicator. If unsuccessful, refer to an ophthalmologist. Once the foreign body has been removed, treat as a corneal abrasion (see Chapter 34).

WHAT IS THE OUTCOME?

Most superficial corneal foreign bodies can be removed with a wet applicator. The residual corneal abrasions resolve within 48 hours.

CHAPTER 36
Conjunctival Foreign Body

WHAT IS IT?

Particulate material, usually airborne, that becomes embedded within the conjunctiva. The favorite resting place is a concavity in the tarsal plate of the upper lid (superior tarsal sulcus).

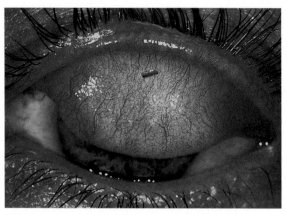

FIGURE 1. Conjunctival foreign body (everted upper lid). The black fragment lies in its favorite resting place: the superior tarsal sulcus.

WHAT DOES IT LOOK LIKE?

The patient complains of a foreign body sensation on blinking, as the foreign body rubs against the cornea. The offending particle—typically black or brown—usually lies in the superior tarsal sulcus. A corneal abrasion may be present.

WHAT ELSE LOOKS LIKE IT?

Nothing.

HOW DO YOU DIAGNOSE?

By linking the symptoms and the conjunctival findings.

HOW DO YOU MANAGE?

Topically anesthetize the affected eye and measure visual acuity. Inspect the cornea and stain with fluorescein to rule out any abrasions. Evert the upper lid, inspect the tarsal sulcus, and remove foreign material with a wet applicator. If unsuccessful, refer to an ophthalmologist. If there is an associated corneal abrasion, treat as you would a corneal abrasion (see Chapter 34). Otherwise no further treatment is needed.

WHAT IS THE OUTCOME?

Most conjunctival foreign bodies are easy to remove. The skill is in learning to evert the upper lid.

CHAPTER 37
Corneal Ulcer

WHAT IS IT?

An erosion of the epithelium and stroma of the cornea; it can be infected or sterile. Infectious causes are bacteria, fungi, protozoans, and herpes simplex. Noninfectious causes include trigeminal denervation (neurotrophic keratitis), severe dry eye syndrome, connective tissue diseases, chemical burn, vernal conjunctivitis, and staphylococcal hypersensitivity.

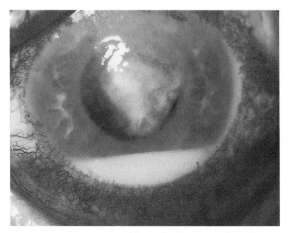

FIGURE 1. Corneal ulcer. The central cornea has a white opacity. Lying at the bottom of the anterior chamber is a layer of pus (hypopyon).

WHAT DOES IT LOOK LIKE?

One or more white patches on the cornea with fuzzy margins. The involved areas may show corneal thinning. The conjunctiva is always hyperemic, especially near the cornea (ciliary flush, circumcorneal injection).

WHAT ELSE LOOKS LIKE IT?

Healed corneal scars. But healed scars do not have fuzzy margins and the conjunctiva is not hyperemic. The patient does not have a foreign body sensation or photophobia.

HOW DO YOU DIAGNOSE?

By the characteristic corneal findings. Scrapings of the ulcer may not yield the causative organisms; in severe cases, and for those unresponsive to empiric therapy, a biopsy is necessary for diagnosis and management.

HOW DO YOU MANAGE?

Refer promptly to an ophthalmologist. Delayed or inappropriate management could lead to severe visual loss.

WHAT IS THE OUTCOME?

Depends on the nature of the lesion, the host, and the timeliness and intensity of treatment. Mild cases may resolve with minimal visual loss. More severe cases may require corneal transplantation or other surgical measures.

CHAPTER 38
Corneoscleral Laceration

WHAT IS IT?

Traumatic rent of the cornea and sclera. It can be caused by a sharp instrument, a missile, or a blow. It can penetrate or perforate the injured tissue.

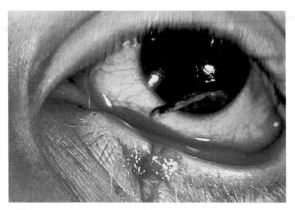

FIGURE 1. Corneoscleral laceration. A cut extends across the inferior cornea and sclera. The iris has prolapsed into the hole.

WHAT DOES IT LOOK LIKE?

A corneal laceration is easier to recognize than a scleral laceration because it disrupts the shape and transparency of the tissue. A scleral laceration can be occult because the overlying conjunctiva is swollen and hemorrhagic. Suspect a ruptured globe if vision is poor, the eye appears misshapen, there is blood in the anterior chamber or vitreous, or the pupil is distorted. Even if these signs are missing, an ophthalmologist will suspect a ruptured globe if the intraocular pressure is very low (below 10 mm Hg).

WHAT ELSE LOOKS LIKE IT?

Severe contusion of the cornea and sclera.

HOW DO YOU DIAGNOSE?

By careful inspection of the eye in a patient with a history of lacerating, contusive, or missile injury.

HOW DO YOU MANAGE?

All but the most superficial corneoscleral lacerations must be surgically repaired under general anesthesia. Repair is urgent to prevent infection.

WHAT IS THE OUTCOME?

Depends on the nature of the injury. Lacerations restricted to the sclera may not cause permanent visual loss unless the retina has been damaged. Small corneal lacerations, particularly those outside the visual axis, may be compatible with adequate visual outcomes. Larger lacerations usually cause enough distortion of vision that transplantation may be necessary.

CHAPTER 39

Chemical Burn

WHAT IS IT?

Chemical contact with the conjunctiva or cornea. Concentrated alkali and acid cause the greatest damage.

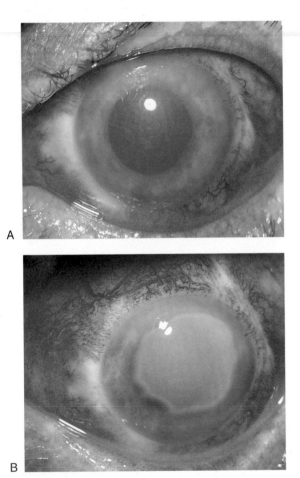

FIGURE 1. Chemical burn. **A:** Acute phase: The cornea is hazy. **B:** Three days later: Fluorescein stains a large epithelial defect.

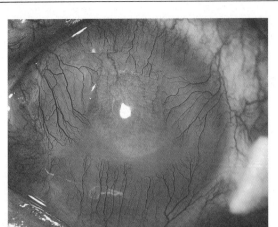

C

FIGURE 1. *Continued.* **C:** Chronic phase: The cornea has been scarred, and conjunctival vessels have grown in.

WHAT DOES IT LOOK LIKE?

If only the conjunctiva has been exposed, the patient complains of stinging. If the cornea has been injured, the patient complains of photophobia and blurred vision. Mild conjunctival injury causes hyperemia; severe injury causes blanching, as the vessels are destroyed. Mild cornea injury is indicated by punctate fluorescein staining; severe corneal injury causes widespread erosion of the epithelium and edema of the stroma. If the chemical is particulate, pieces may be found on the ocular surface and in the conjunctival fornices.

WHAT ELSE LOOKS LIKE IT?

The conjunctival hyperemia of mild chemical exposure can reflect infection or allergy. Severe ocular exposure to toxic chemicals causes unmistakable abnormalities: blanching of the perilimbal conjunctival vessels and clouding of the cornea.

HOW DO YOU DIAGNOSE?

By linking the history and the ocular findings.

HOW DO YOU MANAGE?

Immediately anesthetize the affected eye(s) and undertake copious irrigation with water or balanced salt solution. Specula or retractors are helpful to allow greater exposure. If you suspect particulate chemical exposure, sweep the fornices with a wet applicator to remove retained bits.

Irrigate until litmus paper indicates a neutral pH (7.0). If the conjunctiva is not swollen or blanched and the cornea appears normal with fluorescein, no further treatment is necessary. Otherwise refer immediately to an ophthalmologist.

WHAT IS THE OUTCOME?

Depends on the nature and dose of the chemical that reaches the ocular surface. Alkali and acid burns can devastate the ocular tissues.

C H A P T E R   4 0
Anterior Uveitis

WHAT IS IT?

Inflammation of the iris and ciliary body. It is usually an isolated autoimmune reaction but may be part of a systemic rheumatologic condition such as ankylosing spondylitis, juvenile rheumatoid arthritis, Reiter's syndrome, sarcoidosis, herpes simplex or zoster, or Behçet's disease. (The uveal tract includes the iris, ciliary body, pars plana, and choroid. Anterior uveitis involves the iris and ciliary body; intermediate uveitis involves the pars plana; posterior uveitis involves the choroid.)

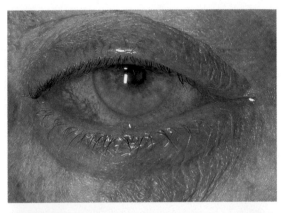

A

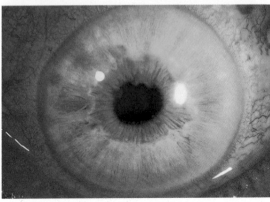

B

FIGURE 1. Anterior uveitis. **A:** Acute phase: dilated conjunctival vessels. **B:** Chronic phase: granulomas on the iris margin. *(continued)*

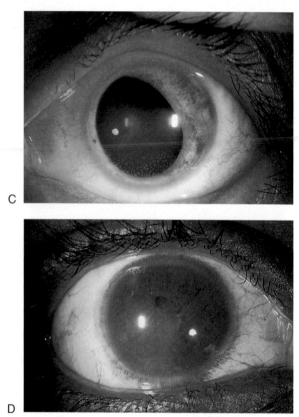

FIGURE 1. Continued. C: Chronic phase: irregularly dilated pupil, reflecting scarring of temporal iris to lens. **D:** Chronic phase: small, irregular pupil, reflecting scarring of iris to lens.

WHAT DOES IT LOOK LIKE?

The patient reports photophobia and pain in the eye and brow. Vision may be blurred but is often normal. The eye shows circumcorneal conjunctival injection (ciliary flush), which is often mild. The pupil may be irregular, reflecting adhesions of the iris to the anterior lens or posterior corneal surface. Slit lamp biomicroscopy reveals turbidity and cellular debris of the aqueous humor; cells may be adherent to the posterior surface of the cornea. Intraocular pressure is usually normal or low.

WHAT ELSE LOOKS LIKE IT?

Keratitis, acute angle closure glaucoma, and episcleritis/scleritis. Keratitis is excluded by the absence of corneal abnormalities after fluorescein staining. Acute angle closure glaucoma usually causes more severe eye pain, the cornea is often slightly turbid, and the intraocular pressure is very high. Episcleritis/scleritis produces conjunctival hyperemia limited to one region rather than a ciliary flush.

HOW DO YOU DIAGNOSE?

By eliciting a history of photophobia without signs of keratitis and by observing cells, flare, and/or iris adhesions with a slit lamp biomicroscope.

HOW DO YOU MANAGE?

Refer to an ophthalmologist because diagnosis and management are difficult. A systemic workup is advisable if the patient has a history suggestive of a rheumatologic illness or if the uveitis is recurrent or resistant to topical therapy.

WHAT IS THE OUTCOME?

Most isolated anterior uveitis resolves without damage either spontaneously or with topical corticosteroid treatment. However, recurrences are common, and some cases become chronic and resistant to therapy. Blindness then becomes a threat.

CHAPTER 41
Acute Angle Closure Glaucoma

WHAT IS IT?

A sudden rise in intraocular pressure consequent to blockage of the aqueous outflow pathway by the iris root. Most attacks occur in otherwise healthy elderly patients whose crystalline lenses are enlarging with age and crowding the anterior chamber. Also at risk are those who have high hyperopia and have had previous ocular inflammation or surgery. (Eyedrops used to dilate the pupil very rarely result in angle closure.)

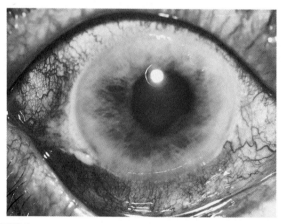

FIGURE 1. Acute angle closure glaucoma. The conjunctival vessels are dilated, especially near the cornea (ciliary flush) and the cornea is translucent (edematous).

WHAT DOES IT LOOK LIKE?

The patient reports sudden excruciating eye or brow pain and blurred vision. The pain may be accompanied by a vagal response, with vomiting and prostration. This reaction often distracts attendants into supposing the problem to be abdominal or intracranial. However, the affected eye is newly red, with ciliary flush and a bedewed cornea. The pupil usually does not react to direct light. Intraocular pressure is very elevated.

WHAT ELSE LOOKS LIKE IT?

Keratitis, uveitis, and episcleritis/scleritis. Keratitis is excluded by the absence of corneal abnormalities after fluorescein staining. Uveitis does not give rise to severe pain, the cornea is usually clear, and intraocular pressure is usually normal. Episcleritis/scleritis produces conjunctival hyperemia limited to one region rather than a ciliary flush.

HOW DO YOU DIAGNOSE?

By linking sudden severe periocular pain to the findings of ciliary flush, cloudy cornea, fixed pupil, and high intraocular pressure. Intraocular pressure should be measured by one of the standard tonometers but can be estimated by digital compression of the eye through closed lids; the affected eye should feel rock hard compared to the unaffected eye.

HOW DO YOU MANAGE?

Refer to an ophthalmologist immediately because sustained elevation of intraocular pressure can seriously damage the optic nerve. If the patient can expect a delay in reaching an ophthalmologist, administer acetazolamide (Diamox) 500 mg i.v. or orally. The ophthalmologist will probably perform a laser iridotomy in an attempt to restore normal aqueous outflow.

WHAT IS THE OUTCOME?

Depends on how extensive the blockage has been. If mild and brief, laser iridotomy is usually successful in restoring normal aqueous flow. Vision usually recovers. But sustained high intraocular pressures will leave permanent optic nerve damage even if outflow is restored. Therefore, acute angle closure glaucoma is an emergency.

Episcleritis/Scleritis

WHAT IS IT?

Autoimmune inflammation of the episclera (episcleritis) or sclera (scleritis). Episcleritis is a vasculitis of the deep conjunctival vessels lying on the superficial sclera that is usually isolated and idiopathic but may occur in rheumatologic illness. Scleritis is a focal inflammation akin to a rheumatoid nodule. More often than episcleritis, it is associated with a rheumatologic illness.

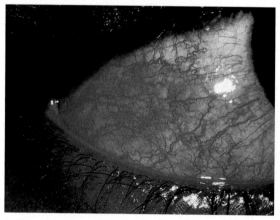

FIGURE 1. Episcleritis. Focal hyperemia and swelling of the conjunctival and underlying episcleral vessels.

WHAT DOES IT LOOK LIKE?

Episcleritis and scleritis cause pain in the eye (mild in episcleritis, more severe in scleritis) and usually a focal hyperemia of the deep conjunctival vessels. In scleritis, the sclera often becomes necrotic and thin, making it look gray or blue as the underlying black choroid shows through.

WHAT ELSE LOOKS LIKE IT?

An inflamed pingueculum, a pterygium, or focal conjunctivitis. An inflamed pingueculum is an idiopathically degenerated area of conjunctiva near the corneal limbus, usually nasal, that may transiently attract vessels and sting. Its center contains a grayish-yellow patch. A ptery-gium is an area of fleshy, hyperemic conjunctiva, usually nasal, that has been activated by sun exposure and grows toward or onto the cornea. It rarely causes much discomfort. Uncommonly, infectious conjunctivitis may be focal.

HOW DO YOU DIAGNOSE?

By discovering an area of focal conjunctival hyperemia that appears to affect very deep vessels and is associated with eye pain. Look for the ominous blue-gray patch that denotes scleral thinning in scleritis. There should be no conjunctival mounding to suggest a pingueculum or pterygium, or discharge to suggest infectious conjunctivitis. Even so, the diagnosis may be difficult.

HOW DO YOU MANAGE?

Refer to an ophthalmologist because diagnosis and management may be difficult. Episcleritis usually responds quickly to topical corticos-teroids or ketorolac. Scleritis is resistant to topical medication, requir-ing systemic corticosteroids or other immunosuppressive agents.

WHAT IS THE OUTCOME?

Most cases of episcleritis usually respond quickly but, like anterior uveitis, it often recurs. Scleritis is always difficult to manage. Vision may be lost owing to involvement of the cornea, choroid, retina, or op-tic nerve.

Endophthalmitis

WHAT IS IT?

Infection of all the internal portions of the eye—the anterior chamber, iris, ciliary body, vitreous, retina, and choroid. If the infection spreads to adjacent orbital tissue, it is called panophthalmitis. It may arise from an entry wound (trauma, intraocular surgery) or from hematogenous sepsis.

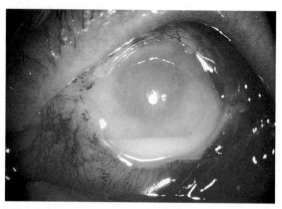

FIGURE 1. Endophthalmitis. Hazy cornea and hypopyon and markedly inflamed conjunctiva.

WHAT DOES IT LOOK LIKE?

The patient has severe eye pain. The lids are swollen, the conjunctiva is hyperemic, the cornea is usually cloudy, and the anterior chamber contains pus, which often layers out as a meniscus (hypopyon). The lens may be visible, but the vitreous is usually so turbid that the retina cannot be seen.

WHAT ELSE LOOKS LIKE IT?

Severe keratitis, anterior uveitis, and angle closure glaucoma. Keratitis and anterior uveitis may cause equivalent pain and a hypopyon but rarely involve the orbital tissues. Angle closure glaucoma never causes a hypopyon and raises intraocular pressure higher than does endophthalmitis.

HOW DO YOU DIAGNOSE?

By finding signs of severe inflammation inside the eye in a setting of eye trauma, surgery, systemic sepsis, or an immunocompromised state. A definite diagnosis is based on aspirating organisms from inside the eye.

HOW DO YOU MANAGE?

Refer immediately to an ophthalmologist because diagnosis and management are difficult. Treatment consists of removing infected vitreous and injecting antibiotics into the eye.

WHAT IS THE OUTCOME?

Most eyes are lost. However, early diagnosis and treatment can be vision saving.

CHAPTER 44

Inflamed Pingueculum

WHAT IS IT?

A fleshy area of nasal or temporal conjunctiva that temporarily becomes mildly painful, swells, and attracts blood vessels. Pathologically, it consists of benign hyperplasia. It may be a mild version of a pterygium (see Chapter 45).

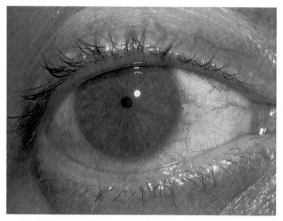

FIGURE 1. Inflamed pingueculum. A small, yellow, gelatinous patch of conjunctiva at the nasal corneal margin attracts vessels.

WHAT DOES IT LOOK LIKE?

A yellow-white patch of conjunctiva surrounded by blood vessels.

WHAT ELSE LOOKS LIKE IT?

Pterygium, conjunctival neoplasms. A pterygium is a wing-shaped mound of fibrovascular tissue that grows toward or onto the cornea. Conjunctival neoplasms, usually squamous, differ by lack of pain and by steady, concentric growth.

HOW DO YOU DIAGNOSE?

By its characteristic appearance and the regression of surrounding vessels within days of treatment with topical corticosteroids or ketorolac.

HOW DO YOU MANAGE?

If the lesion is distinctive, treat with topical corticosteroid (prednisolone 1/8%) or ketorolac for 1 week. If there is no response, or if the lesion recurs, refer to an ophthalmologist.

WHAT IS THE OUTCOME?

Most inflamed pinguecula retreat to small, avascular, yellow-white mounds within days of topical therapy. Recurrences are uncommon.

CHAPTER 45
Pterygium

WHAT IS IT?

A benign fibrovascular conjunctival lesion that starts in the nasal or temporal area and grows toward or onto the cornea. Occurring commonly in persons exposed to sunlight, it is considered an actinic hyperplasia. Once it reaches the cornea, it distorts and obscures vision.

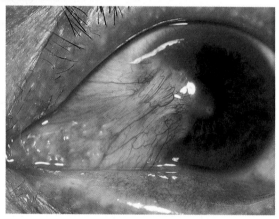

FIGURE 1. Pterygium. "Winged" growth of hyperplastic conjunctiva onto the cornea.

WHAT DOES IT LOOK LIKE?

A triangular (wing-shaped) frond with its apex aimed at the cornea.

WHAT ELSE LOOKS LIKE IT?

A conjunctival dermoid, a papilloma, a neoplasm, or previous eye surgery or trauma. The winged shape, its apex toward the cornea, is distinctive.

HOW DO YOU DIAGNOSE?

By its characteristic appearance.

HOW DO YOU MANAGE?

A pterygium does not respond to medication. Unless it is distorting or obscuring the cornea, it requires no treatment. Otherwise, surgical removal is necessary.

WHAT IS THE OUTCOME?

Pterygia usually grow, but sometimes very slowly. Surgical removal often improves vision, but regrowth is common.

CHAPTER 46
Subconjunctival Hemorrhage

WHAT IS IT?

An area of extravascular blood within the conjunctiva. Apart from trauma (including childbirth), it occurs most often in the elderly, whose friable vessels burst during a sneeze or other strain. It also happens in systemic hypertension and bleeding disorders.

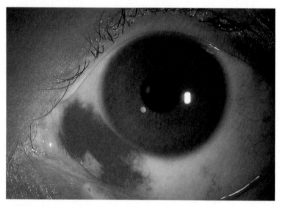

FIGURE 1. Subconjunctival hemorrhage. Extravasated blood in the inferior conjunctiva.

WHAT DOES IT LOOK LIKE?

One or more patches of red overlying the sclera.

WHAT ELSE LOOKS LIKE IT?

Conjunctival hyperemia. But dilated blood vessels should be easy to differentiate from one or more patches of extravascular blood.

HOW DO YOU DIAGNOSE?

By its characteristic appearance.

Subconjunctival Hemorrhage

HOW DO YOU MANAGE?

Unless there is a persuasive history of trauma or strain, rule out hypertension and bleeding disorders.

WHAT IS THE OUTCOME?

The blood disappears completely within weeks. During this time, the conjunctiva becomes temporarily discolored yellow by blood breakdown products.

CHAPTER 47

Iris Melanoma

WHAT IS IT?

A malignancy of iris melanocytes. If isolated to the iris, it is considered a very low threat to metastasize. If it is an anterior extension of a ciliary body melanoma, the prognosis is worse.

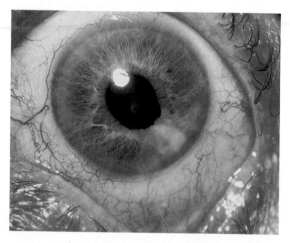

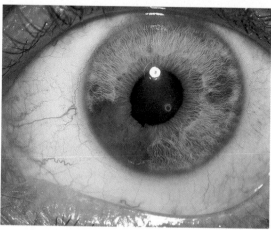

FIGURE 1. Iris melanoma. A variety of pigmented growths on the iris.

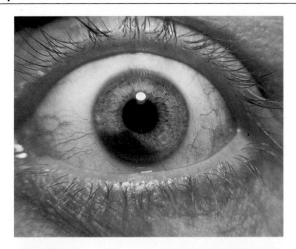

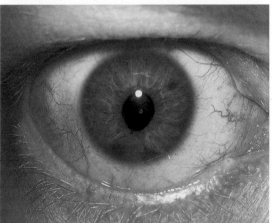

FIGURE 1. *Continued*

WHAT DOES IT LOOK LIKE?

A brown or gray mound on the iris. It may distort the pupil. Many months must elapse before growth is evident.

WHAT ELSE LOOKS LIKE IT?

An iris nevus, which is far more common. Nevi do not usually grow. Otherwise there is no easy way to distinguish the appearance of nevi from that of melanomas.

HOW DO YOU DIAGNOSE?

Appearance does not allow you to distinguish a melanoma from a nevus. Growth indicates a melanoma. A definite diagnosis depends on a biopsy.

HOW DO YOU MANAGE?

By documenting growth and then excising.

WHAT IS THE OUTCOME?

Iris melanomas are usually low grade and cured by excision.

CHAPTER 48
Anisocoria

WHAT IS IT?

A difference in diameter between the two pupils. Unless the difference is greater than 1 mm, anisocoria is probably not pathologic. Pathologic anisocoria may result from a lesion of the parasympathetic pathway (mediated by the third cranial nerve), the sympathetic pathway, eyedrops, or trauma or inflammation of the iris itself.

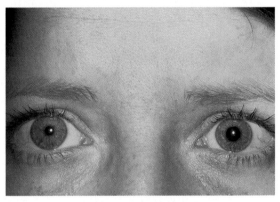

FIGURE 1. Anisocoria. Pupil diameters in the two eyes are visibly different.

WHAT DOES IT LOOK LIKE?

A difference in pupil size in the dimmest illumination that allows observation.

WHAT ELSE LOOKS LIKE IT?

Nothing.

HOW DO YOU DIAGNOSE?

By observing the pupil size difference in very dim light. Determining the cause is more difficult. Assess pupil reactivity to direct light, to a near target, and note pertinent associated signs (ptosis, ocular motility abnormalities).

HOW DO YOU MANAGE?

Depends on the cause. Refer to an ophthalmologist if you suspect pathologic anisocoria, particularly if the finding is recent.

WHAT IS THE OUTCOME?

Depends on the cause.

CHAPTER 49

Traumatic Hyphema

WHAT IS IT?

Bleeding in the anterior chamber of the eye. Nearly all cases are caused by direct trauma to the globe. The bleeding results from a tear in a blood vessel at the iris root and suggests substantial contusion of the eye. Hyphema may be isolated or may be part of other injuries to the eye.

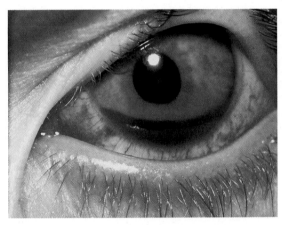

FIGURE 1. Traumatic hyphema. A layer of blood at the bottom of the anterior chamber.

WHAT DOES IT LOOK LIKE?

A meniscus of dark-red blood layered at the bottom of the anterior chamber. In the worst case, blood fills the entire chamber, making the eye look like a red billiard ball. The intraocular pressure may be very elevated, as blood blocks the egress of aqueous. The patient complains of blurred vision and often eye pain, the result of contusion of the anterior uvea or elevated intraocular pressure.

WHAT ELSE LOOKS LIKE IT?

Nothing.

HOW DO YOU DIAGNOSE?

By its characteristic appearance.

HOW DO YOU MANAGE?

Refer to an ophthalmologist. Patients who have no other injuries and whose intraocular pressure is normal can be managed on bed rest with eye shielding. More troublesome cases require hospitalization, sometimes including surgical evacuation of the blood.

WHAT IS THE OUTCOME?

Uncomplicated, mild hyphemas usually resolve spontaneously within days. However, they often reflect other damage to the eye that may cause permanent vision loss.

Cataract

WHAT IS IT?

Opacification of the eye's crystalline lens. Aging, ocular trauma, inflammation, and metabolic dysfunction are the principal causes.

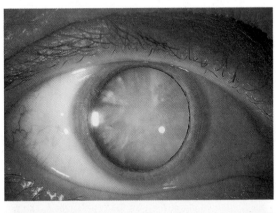

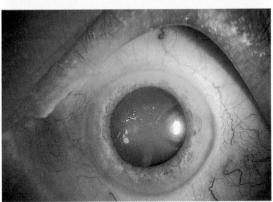

FIGURE 1. Cataract. **A:** Dense cataract (lens opacity). **B:** Sparkling opacities in an early cataract.

WHAT DOES IT LOOK LIKE?

An early cataract may be hard to detect without a slit lamp biomicroscope. As the opacification increases, the red reflex visible through a direct ophthalmoscope becomes dim or dull. Finally the red reflex disappears altogether. With an extremely dense cataract, the pupil turns from black to white (leukocoria).

WHAT ELSE LOOKS LIKE IT?

The red reflex can be lost when the vitreous becomes cloudy (hemorrhage, inflammation, scar) or if the retina is tumorous or detached.

HOW DO YOU DIAGNOSE?

By finding subnormal visual acuity and an altered red reflex. Ophthalmologists use a combination of slit lamp biomicroscopy and ophthalmoscopy to confirm the diagnosis.

HOW DO YOU MANAGE?

By referring to an ophthalmologist who will extract the cataract if it is impairing vision. Most cataract surgery is now done by incising the lens capsule, fragmenting the cataract with an ultrasonic device, removing the fragments by suction, and replacing the crystalline lens with a plastic lens implanted within the capsular bag. The posterior lens capsule may later opacify, but this can usually be rectified with laser treatment.

WHAT IS THE OUTCOME?

Modern cataract surgery offers full restoration of distance vision in nearly all cases, provided the other parts of the eye are functioning normally. Complications occur in fewer than 2% of cases, and they are rarely visually debilitating.

CHAPTER 51
Dislocated Lens

WHAT IS IT?

Slippage of the eye's crystalline lens out of its normal position. If the displacement is minor, the patient may not notice any loss of vision. A more drastic shift usually disturbs vision and may cause other problems, such as inflammation or glaucoma. Apart from trauma, the most common causes are Marfan's syndrome and homocystinuria.

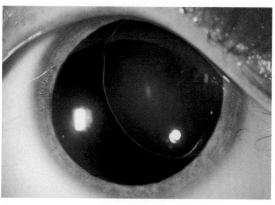

FIGURE 1. Dislocated lens. Inferior lens margin is visible with the dilated pupil. The lens is upwardly and outwardly dislocated.

WHAT DOES IT LOOK LIKE?

Minor displacements are not visible, especially without a slit lamp or with the pupils dilated. Major forward displacements are visible because they distort the pupil. Lateral displacements may reveal the edge of the lens through the pupil. Posterior displacements are suggested by abnormal fluttering of the iris (iridodonesis) and are visible with biomicroscopy and ophthalmoscopy.

WHAT ELSE LOOKS LIKE IT?

Nothing.

HOW DO YOU DIAGNOSE?

With slit lamp biomicroscopy and ophthalmoscopy.

HOW DO YOU MANAGE?

Dislocated lenses are left alone unless they interfere with vision, cause glaucoma, or rub against the inside of the cornea.

WHAT IS THE OUTCOME?

Depends on the position of the lens and the condition of the other parts of the eye.

CHAPTER 52

Vitreous Hemorrhage

WHAT IS IT?

Bleeding into the vitreous cavity. The bleeding comes from torn or incompetent retinal vessels. Apart from trauma, the common causes are diabetes mellitus, hypertension, and bleeding disorders.

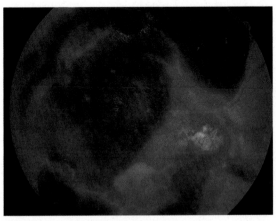

FIGURE 1. Vitreous hemorrhage. Clumped blood in the vitreous obscures view of the retina. (Courtesy of WFUEC.)

WHAT DOES IT LOOK LIKE?

The patient reports acute, painless, blurred or blotchy vision. The red reflex turns dark. Through the ophthalmoscope, the retina is obscured. Dark clumps may be visible within the vitreous.

WHAT ELSE LOOKS LIKE IT?

Cataract, vitreous inflammation, retinal tumor or inflammation. Differentiating among these causes demands the use of a slit lamp biomicroscope and skilled ophthalmoscopy.

HOW DO YOU DIAGNOSE?

By its characteristic appearance.

HOW DO YOU MANAGE?

Depends on the cause.

WHAT IS THE OUTCOME?

Depends on the cause.

CHAPTER 53

Vitreous Inflammation

WHAT IS IT?

Infectious or noninfectious inflammation of the vitreous cavity. The source of the inflammation is either the retina or the choroid. Although some cases are idiopathic, an uncomfortably large number of patients have vision-threatening and life-threatening systemic illnesses that are difficult to manage.

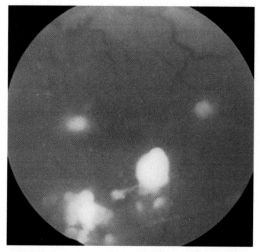

FIGURE 1. Vitreous inflammation. White opacities consist of candidal granulomas ("fungus balls").

WHAT DOES IT LOOK LIKE?

The patient reports a slow onset of blurred vision, often dotted with floaters. The red reflex becomes dull or dark. Biomicroscopy and ophthalmoscopy disclose cells suspended within the vitreous gel, and often an underlying retinal or choroidal disorder.

WHAT ELSE LOOKS LIKE IT?

Vitreous hemorrhage.

HOW DO YOU DIAGNOSE?

By its characteristic appearance.

HOW DO YOU MANAGE?

Depends on the cause.

WHAT IS THE OUTCOME?

Depends on the cause.

CHAPTER 54

Vitreous Detachment

WHAT IS IT?

Separation of the vitreous from the retinal surface. A natural consequence of aging, vitreous detachment usually occurs in the sixties or seventies. It usually goes unnoticed, but sometimes a portion of the posterior vitreous overlying the macula is dense enough to block vision as a floater. It may gradually settle out of view or remain as an annoying obstruction. In rare cases, the detaching vitreous may pull off a piece of retina. If this happens, the retina can detach and drastically impair vision. Retinal detachment is a surgical emergency.

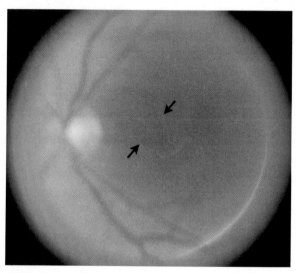

FIGURE 1. Vitreous detachment. The faint ring in the center (*arrows*) is a condensation of the vitreous that has detached from the anterior surface of the retina. It appeared as a ringlike floater to the patient.

WHAT DOES IT LOOK LIKE?

The patient suddenly sees a black or gray fleck, cobweb, or ring floating in the center or edge of the visual field. The floater moves as the eye shifts its gaze, but the floater's movement lags behind the eye movement.

WHAT ELSE LOOKS LIKE IT?

Vitreous hemorrhage or inflammation.

HOW DO YOU DIAGNOSE?

By its characteristic appearance. But skilled ophthalmoscopy is necessary to see it.

HOW DO YOU MANAGE?

If there is no retinal break or detachment, no treatment is necessary. Advise the patient to seek attention if more floaters or further blurring of vision occurs (possibly a symptom of retinal detachment).

WHAT IS THE OUTCOME?

Depends on the cause.

CHAPTER 55

Retinal Detachment

WHAT IS IT?

A separation of the two leaves of the retina. Retinal detachment usually results from a tear in the inner leaf of the retina that occurs when the vitreous gel forcefully detaches. The vitreous gel develops water pockets with age, inflammation, ocular trauma, or surgery. The water pockets make the vitreous unstable and put tension on vitreoretinal attachments. If vitreous detachment also tears off a piece of retina, the liquid vitreous will seep through the retina hole and pry the two leaves of retina apart (see Fig. 1). Visual transmission is blocked through the detached portion and the patient becomes blind in that field.

WHAT DOES IT LOOK LIKE?

The patient complains of suddenly seeing flashing lights and, sometimes, black flecks, then noticing an area of blurred or absent vision (scotoma). The flashes come from vitreous tugging on the retina and stimulating retinal photoreceptors. The flecks, or floaters, come from the vitreous bleeding that results from a retinal vessel torn by the de-

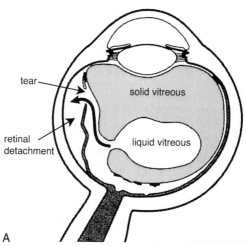

A

FIGURE 1. Retinal detachment. **A:** Schematic cross-section of the eye shows that a contracting vitreous has torn a hole in the peripheral retina; liquid vitreous pours through the hole and separates (detaches) the two leaves of a portion of the retina. *(continued)*

119

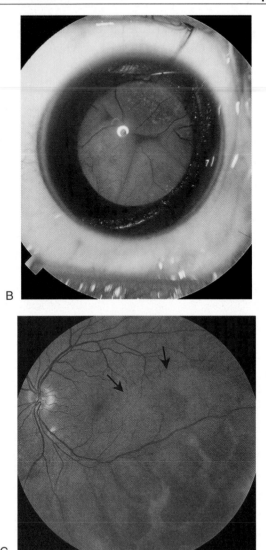

FIGURE 1. *Continued.* **B:** (picture taken through pupil) Ballooned detached retina is visible through the pupil. Retinal detachment is rarely so obvious! **C:** (fundus photo) Inferior retinal detachment is visible as rounded elevation with its margin encroaching on the fovea *(arrows)*.

tachment. The scotoma comes from the non-functioning detached retina. Visual acuity may be normal if the detachment does not extend to the fovea. Pupillary reactions are often normal. Retinal detachment is difficult to see with the direct ophthalmoscope because the detachment usually begins in the retinal periphery and may not extend to the optic disc and foveal regions. However, careful dilated ophthalmoscopic examination will disclose that a portion of the normally flat retinal surface now has a ballooned appearance.

WHAT ELSE LOOKS LIKE IT?

Retinal or vitreous inflammation or choroidal tumor. Experienced ophthalmologists can usually make the distinction.

HOW DO YOU DIAGNOSE?

By indirect ophthalmoscopy, sometimes combined with ultrasound.

HOW DO YOU MANAGE?

With surgery. The holes must be located and sealed with cryotherapy applied to the sclera, and the vitreous traction relieved by either removing it or tightening the sclera with encircling plastic bands.

WHAT IS THE OUTCOME?

Depends on the underlying pathology and the duration and extent of the detachment. Retinal detachment is a surgical emergency; the sooner the retina is reattached, the more likely vision can be recovered.

CHAPTER 56
Diabetic Retinopathy

WHAT IS IT?

A disorder of retinal blood vessels that leads to serous leakage, bleeding, and neovascularization. How diabetes causes these vascular changes is still unknown. Their prevalence is much lower when blood sugar is tightly controlled.

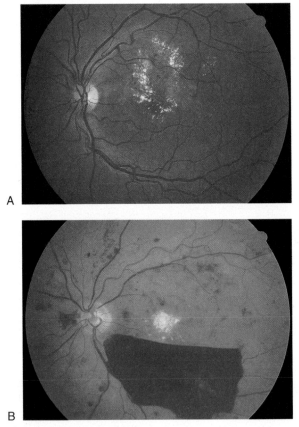

FIGURE 1. Diabetic retinopathy. **A:** Nonproliferative (background). Note the yellow exudates and pinpoint hemorrhages. They reflect microvascular leakage. **B:** Advanced nonproliferative. The hemorrhages and exudates are larger and more numerous.

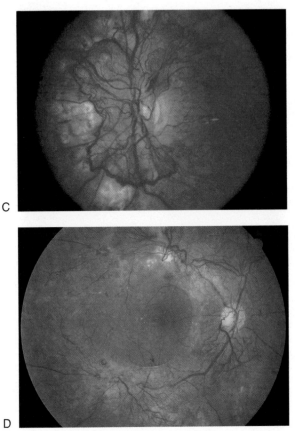

FIGURE 1. *Continued.* C: Proliferative retinopathy. A large net of new blood vessels spans the retinal surface. **D:** A fibrovascular frond elevates the posterior retina. (Courtesy of WFUEC.)

The first stage, called nonproliferative or background retinopathy, consists of capillary microaneurysms, serous leakage, hard exudates, and hemorrhages. At this stage, vision is often normal unless a great deal of serum accumulates within the macula. The second stage, called proliferative retinopathy, consists of neovascularization on the retinal surface. If unchecked, it often leads to massive vitreous hemorrhage and retinal detachment.

WHAT DOES IT LOOK LIKE?

Nonproliferative retinopathy is marked by yellow (hard) exudates and dot and blot hemorrhages scattered around the optic disk and macula. Proliferative retinopathy consists of a net of new blood vessels on the optic disk or nearby. In advanced proliferative retinopathy, the retinal landmarks may be obscured by vitreous hemorrhage and by fibrovascular fronds that extend from the retina into the vitreous cavity.

WHAT ELSE LOOKS LIKE IT?

Nonproliferative diabetic retinopathy can be mimicked by central retinal vein occlusion, retinal vascular malformation, and systemic bleeding or hypertensive disorders. Proliferative retinopathy can be mimicked by ocular trauma or chorioretinal inflammations.

HOW DO YOU DIAGNOSE?

By its characteristic appearance.

HOW DO YOU MANAGE?

By urging strict blood sugar control. Nonproliferative retinopathy is not directly treated unless there is clinically significant macular edema, in which case laser burns are applied in the macular region. Early proliferative retinopathy is treated with laser burns scattered across the entire peripheral retina (panretinal photocoagulation). Advanced proliferative retinopathy requires surgical removal of the vitreous gel (vitrectomy). Collaborative trials have convincingly demonstrated that these treatments significantly improve visual outcome.

WHAT IS THE OUTCOME?

Tight blood sugar control and early photocoagulation treatment reduce vision loss by at least 50%. Because most nonproliferative retinopathy causes no visual symptoms, periodic ophthalmic screening is critical to prevent disabling visual loss.

CHAPTER 57
Hypertensive Retinopathy

WHAT IS IT?

Retinal vasculopathy caused by systemic hypertension. In acute hypertension, retinal arterioles leak serum and blood. If the blood elevation is extreme, the vessels undergo fibrinoid necrosis and portions of the retina become infarcted. In chronic hypertension, the blood vessel walls thicken, become shiny and tortuous, and compress crossing veins. Occlusion of retinal arterioles and veins is a threat.

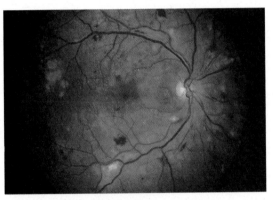

FIGURE 1. Hypertensive retinopathy. Multiple hemorrhages and cotton wool spots. The optic disk is edematous.

WHAT DOES IT LOOK LIKE?

Acute hypertension causes hard exudates, hemorrhages, cotton wool spots (microinfarcts), and large patches of retinal clouding (regional infarcts). Chronic hypertension causes arteriolar walls to glisten with a copper or silver color ("copper wiring," "silver wiring") and to indent and displace crossing veins (arteriovenous nicking).

WHAT ELSE LOOKS LIKE IT?

Nonproliferative diabetic retinopathy, central retinal vein occlusion, and retinal vascular malformations.

HOW DO YOU DIAGNOSE?

By its characteristic appearance.

HOW DO YOU MANAGE?

By controlling blood pressure.

WHAT IS THE OUTCOME?

Blood pressure control usually reverses the leakage and hemorrhage, but infarcted retina does not regenerate.

CHAPTER 58
Embolic Retinopathy

WHAT IS IT?

Embolic particles embedded within retinal arterioles. Most of them originate from the cervical carotid artery bifurcation and are made of platelets and fibrin (Hollenhorst plaques). Sometimes they totally occlude the vessel and cause retinal infarction. But most often they only partially block blood flow and are found incidentally or after transient monocular visual loss. Retinal emboli may also consist of calcium and originate in heart valves.

WHAT DOES IT LOOK LIKE?

A yellow or white spot at the bifurcation of retinal vessels anywhere in the optic fundus. If the retina has been infarcted, a patch of cloudy edema will be seen distal to the embolus.

WHAT ELSE LOOKS LIKE IT?

Retinal vasculitis, which manifests a whitish cuff around vessel segments. But vasculitis affects retinal veins more commonly than arteri-

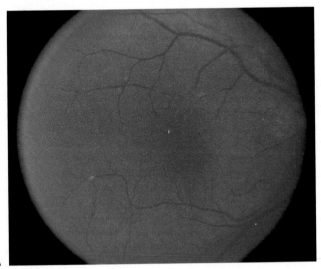

A

FIGURE 1. Embolic retinopathy. **A:** Tiny yellow-white dots are impacted in terminal retinal arterioles. *(continued)*

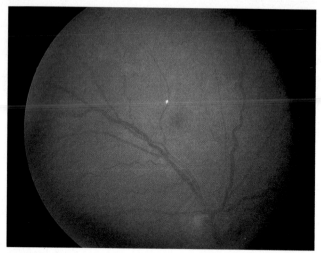

B

FIGURE 1. *Continued.* **B:** A single bright, white dot in a retinal arteriole. (Courtesy of WFUEC.)

oles. Yellow-white patches could also be retinal drusen, hard exudates, or cotton wool spots.

HOW DO YOU DIAGNOSE?

By its characteristic appearance.

HOW DO YOU MANAGE?

By looking for an embolic source—the cervical carotid artery, aortic arch, or heart.

WHAT IS THE OUTCOME?

In most cases, the source is the carotid artery bifurcation, and imaging usually shows atherostenosis or ulceration. The heart is an unlikely source except for calcific aortic stenosis. In at least 30% of cases, no source is found.

CHAPTER 59

Retinal Artery Occlusion

WHAT IS IT?

Blockage of the central retinal artery or one of its branches with infarction of the retina in the domain of the occluded vessel. The cause is local thrombosis (arteriosclerosis, a hypercoagulable state) or an embolism from the cervical carotid artery, aortic arch, or heart.

WHAT DOES IT LOOK LIKE?

The patient complains of a sudden, painless loss of vision in the affected eye. Depending on the extent of the infarct, visual acuity loss may be mild or severe, and visual field defects may be limited or widespread. The infarcted retina loses its transparency and becomes cloudy gray-white (ischemic edema). If the macular region is affected, there will be a cherry-red spot in the fovea. This is because the foveal retina is not infarcted, as it is nourished by the choroidal rather than the retinal arterioles. If the vascular occlusion is embolic, a yellow-white plaque may be visible in the blocked vessel.

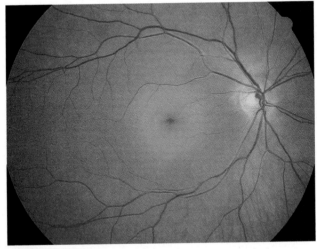

A

FIGURE 1. Retinal artery occlusion. **A:** Central retinal artery occlusion. The central retina is cloudy white (infarcted), and there is a cherry-red spot in the fovea. *(continued)*

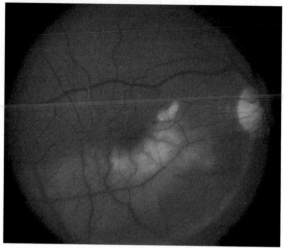

B

FIGURE 1. *Continued.* B: Branch retinal artery occlusion. The inferior temporal arteriole is occluded, causing a cloudy-white area of infarcted retina.

WHAT ELSE LOOKS LIKE IT?

Retinal detachment or inflammation. In retinal detachment, the retina billows forward as liquid vitreous seeps under it. In retinal inflammation [cytomegalovirus (CMV) retinitis, toxoplasmosis], the areas of necrosis are patchy and the overlying vitreous is usually cloudy.

HOW DO YOU DIAGNOSE?

By its characteristic appearance.

HOW DO YOU MANAGE?

There is no known effective treatment for retinal infarction. Intraarterial thrombolysis is of unproved value and is currently performed only for infarcts of less than 4 hours' duration in a patient whose other eye is blind. If a proximal embolus is seen, it is customary to massage the eye in hopes of lowering intraocular pressure enough to dislodge it.

Otherwise, management consists of hunting for an embolic source and modifying arteriosclerotic risk factors.

WHAT IS THE OUTCOME?

In most cases, some recovery of vision occurs within weeks, as the ischemic penumbra recovers. But many patients are left with woeful sight. An embolic source is often not found, especially in central retinal artery occlusion, which may reflect local thrombosis.

CHAPTER 60

Retinal Vein Occlusion

WHAT IS IT?

Blockage of the central retinal vein or one of its tributaries. The cause is usually presumed to be arteriosclerosis. Less commonly, patients have a hypercoagulable state or an orbital mass lesion.

WHAT DOES IT LOOK LIKE?

The patient reports sudden, painless loss of vision in the affected eye. Sometimes the visual loss is preceded or accompanied by flickering lights (scintillations). If the central retinal vein has been occluded, the entire retina will be covered with blotchy, flame-shaped hemorrhages, as if grazed by a red paintbrush. The hemorrhages may be limited to a retinal segment if the occlusion has affected only a branch retinal vein.

WHAT ELSE LOOKS LIKE IT?

Hypertensive and diabetic retinopathy and cytomegalovirus (CMV) retinitis.

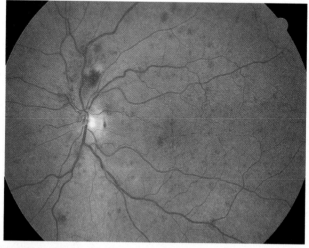

A

FIGURE 1. Retinal vein occlusion. **A:** Mild central retinal vein occlusion. Dilated retinal veins and scattered perivenous hemorrhages.

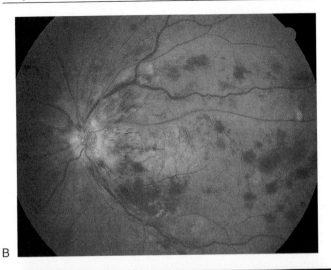

B

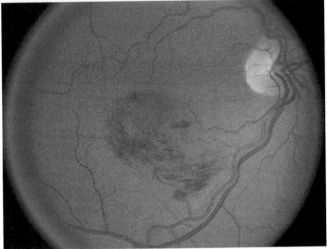

C

FIGURE 1. *Continued.* B: Marked central retinal vein occlusion. The retina is covered with surface hemorrhages from exploded veins. **C:** Branch retinal vein occlusion. The inferior temporal branch is occluded, causing hemorrhage in that region. (Courtesy of WFUEC.)

133

HOW DO YOU DIAGNOSE?

By its characteristic appearance.

HOW DO YOU MANAGE?

There is no acute treatment for retinal vein occlusion. But these patients require monitoring by an ophthalmologist because some will later develop neovascular glaucoma and others will develop persistent macular edema that must be treated with laser photocoagulation.

WHAT IS THE OUTCOME?

Depends on the extent of the occlusion. The worst cases end up with severe visual loss. The milder cases often show remarkable spontaneous recovery. Vision improves as blood and edema resolve.

CHAPTER 61

Cotton Wool Spot

WHAT IS IT?

A retinal microinfarct caused by occlusion of a precapillary arteriole. Pathologically, it consists of dilated retinal ganglion cell axons whose axoplasm has been focally arrested.

A myriad of conditions may produce a cotton wool spot: diabetes mellitus, systemic hypertension, human immunodeficiency virus (HIV), connective tissue disease, blood dyscrasia, altitude sickness, ocular exposure to x-irradiation, intravenous drug abuse, trauma with chest compression or long bone fractures, pancreatitis, sepsis, and spirochetal and rickettsial diseases.

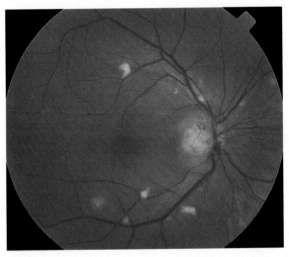

FIGURE 1. Cotton wool spots. Multiple feathery white spots on the retina. They signify microinfarcts of the retinal nerve fiber layer. (Courtesy of WFUEC.)

WHAT DOES IT LOOK LIKE?

A feathery white patch on the retina that covers its surface vessels. There may be one or many cotton wool spots, their long axes aimed at the optic disk. Patients usually do not notice any visual disturbance unless the cotton wool spots are numerous or located next to the fovea.

WHAT ELSE LOOKS LIKE IT?

Retinal drusen, myelinated retinal nerve fibers, hard exudates, and retinal infiltrates. Retinal drusen are waxy yellow rather than white and are concentrated around the fovea. Myelinated retinal nerve fibers are larger and are connected to the optic disk. Hard exudates are yellow, have more discrete margins, and are not radially oriented to the optic disk. Retinal infiltrates are larger and usually have an overlying vitreous haze.

HOW DO YOU DIAGNOSE?

By its characteristic appearance.

HOW DO YOU MANAGE?

By searching for the underlying cause.

WHAT IS THE OUTCOME?

Depends on the cause.

Cytomegalovirus Retinopathy

WHAT IS IT?

Infection of the retina by cytomegalovirus (CMV). The infection starts with necrotic occlusion of retinal arterioles and spreads like fire across the retina, leaving liquefactive and hemorrhagic destruction in its path.

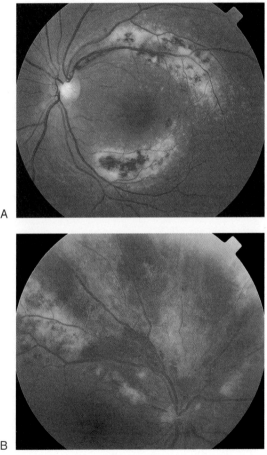

FIGURE 1. Cytomegalovirus retinitis. **A:** Early stage. Hemorrhagic necrosis along the temporal vascular arcades. **B:** Advanced stage. Hemorrhagic necrosis of the upper half of the retina. (Courtesy of WFUEC.)

WHAT DOES IT LOOK LIKE?

In the beginning, there may be one or more patches of whitish infiltrates in the macular region or in the peripheral retina. Within days to weeks, the patches enlarge along blood vessel routes and become speckled with hemorrhages.

WHAT ELSE LOOKS LIKE IT?

Cotton wool spots, retinal vein occlusion, other herpesvirus retinal infections.

HOW DO YOU DIAGNOSE?

By its characteristic appearance and time course. In the initial stage, it may be difficult to distinguish from a cotton wool spot. In later stages it is difficult to separate it from retinitis caused by herpes simplex or zoster. CMV retinitis is usually a part of systemic CMV infection, and other involved sites are soon found.

HOW DO YOU MANAGE?

With intravenous or intraocular ganciclovir or foscarnet. Ganciclovir-containing implants can be sewn onto the inner wall of the sclera. Such local treatment is highly effective in arresting the retinitis and avoids the systemic toxicity of parenteral antiviral therapy.

WHAT IS THE OUTCOME?

Depends on the patient's immune status and on whether the retinitis is diagnosed before extensive damage has occurred.

CHAPTER 63
Age-Related Macular Degeneration

WHAT IS IT?

An idiopathic degeneration of the retina in the macular region. The most common cause of vision loss among the elderly, it is usually slowly progressive and binocular, although the two eyes may be asymmetrically affected. In some cases, visual loss is acute, as blood dissects under the retina from a vascular membrane that originates in the choroid.

WHAT DOES IT LOOK LIKE?

The dry form of macular degeneration, which accounts for more than 90% of cases, produces waxy yellow spots called drusen. Drusen are elastic mounds that mark the regions where the retinal pigment epithelium has died. When drusen become confluent, visual acuity fails. The much rarer wet form of macular degeneration accounts for the most severe visual loss in this condition. A choroidal vascular membrane burrows into the macula; its fragile vessels eventually bleed and disrupt the photoreceptors.

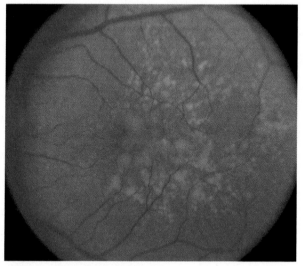

A

FIGURE 1. Age-related macular degeneration. **A:** Dry form. Multiple gray-white spots called drusen fill the foveal region; they reflect the death of pigment epithelium there. *(continued)*

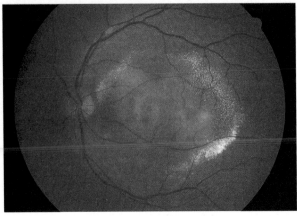

B

FIGURE 1. *Continued.* **B:** Wet form. The foveal region is discolored gray and yellow. This reflects bleeding under the retina caused by choroidal neovascularization.

WHAT ELSE LOOKS LIKE IT?

Rarer conditions that affect the macular region, such as toxoplasmosis, dystrophies, and toxicity from sun gazing or excessive chloroquine ingestion.

HOW DO YOU DIAGNOSE?

By its characteristic appearance.

HOW DO YOU MANAGE?

There is no treatment for the dry form. The wet form is sometimes treated with laser photocoagulation, which retards visual loss but does not restore vision. Patients may have to be trained to use vision-enhancing optical devices.

WHAT IS THE OUTCOME?

The dry form causes inexorable visual acuity loss, but it may be mild or very slowly progressive. The wet form can produce sudden, devastating visual acuity loss, which is why laser photocoagulation of an early choroidal vascular membrane may be critical.

CHAPTER 64

Sickle Retinopathy

WHAT IS IT?

Retinopathy caused by occlusion of retinal vessels by sickling erythrocytes. The findings occur first in the peripheral retina, where vessels have a narrow caliber. They consist of new vessel formation, hemorrhage, and retinal detachment. These findings are common in sickle-C and sickle-Thal, uncommon in SS, and rare in AS.

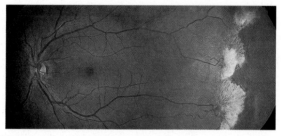

FIGURE 1. Sickle cell retinopathy. Peripheral retinal vessels form fanlike structures in an attempt to vascularize hypoxic retina. (Courtesy of WFUEC.)

WHAT DOES IT LOOK LIKE?

Subhyaloid hemorrhages and neovascular tufts appear in the peripheral retina, out of view of a direct ophthalmoscope. Therefore, patients can harbor vision-threatening retinopathy that is asymptomatic and visible only with special optical instruments.

WHAT ELSE LOOKS LIKE IT?

Retinopathy of prematurity.

HOW DO YOU DIAGNOSE?

By its characteristic appearance.

HOW DO YOU MANAGE?

Some patients require laser photocoagulation or cryotherapy of the peripheral retinal pathology.

WHAT IS THE OUTCOME?

Depends on whether the disease is caught early. Once it is advanced, visual loss may be irreversible.

CHAPTER 65

Retinopathy of Blood Dyscrasias

WHAT IS IT?

Retinopathy caused by anemia, thrombocytopenia, polycythemia, or leukemia. These conditions all cause retinal vascular occlusion, microinfarcts, and bleeding.

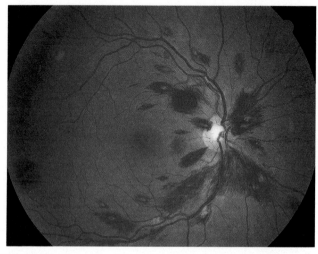

FIGURE 1. Retinopathy of blood dyscrasia. Retinal hemorrhages and white-centered hemorrhages (Roth spots), reflecting ischemia and vascular incompetence from severe anemia and thrombocytopenia in a patient with acute myeloblastic leukemia. (Courtesy of WFUEC.)

WHAT DOES IT LOOK LIKE?

Cotton wool spots and hemorrhages (dot-, blot-, flame-, boat-shaped).

WHAT ELSE LOOKS LIKE IT?

Diabetic, hypertensive, and x-irradiation retinopathy.

HOW DO YOU DIAGNOSE?

By linking the retinal findings to abnormalities on examination of venous blood.

HOW DO YOU MANAGE?

By correcting the blood dyscrasia.

WHAT IS THE OUTCOME?

Most retinal abnormalities resolve within weeks to months of correction of the blood dyscrasia.

CHAPTER 66

Toxoplasmic Retinitis

WHAT IS IT?

Granulomatous retinal infiltration by the encysted form of the parasite *Toxoplasma gondii*. The infection is usually acquired in utero from an infected mother. The retina is among many central nervous system sites that may be seeded. The granulomas can be quiescent for a lifetime and discovered only incidentally. However, dying organisms may excite inflammation that degrades vision.

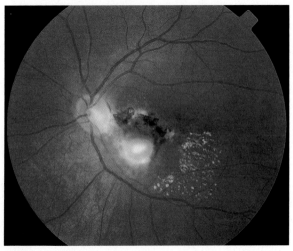

FIGURE 1. Toxoplasmic retinitis. Cloudy-white spot at lower edge of black pigmented retinal scar and nearby hard, yellow exudates reflect reactivation of a congenital toxoplasmic lesion. (Courtesy of WFUEC.)

WHAT DOES IT LOOK LIKE?

The quiescent form displays a round chorioretinal scar that typically has a white center and a black border. The activated form consists of a fuzzy white patch with an overlying vitreous haze ("headlight in a fog"). It is generally adjacent to a quiescent scar. Because most lesions are located in or near the fovea, visual acuity is at risk.

WHAT ELSE LOOKS LIKE IT?

Retinitis caused by *Candida* organisms, *Toxocara canis*, syphilis, and cytomegalovirus (CMV).

HOW DO YOU DIAGNOSE?

By its characteristic appearance and the finding of elevated immunoglobulins specific to the organism.

HOW DO YOU MANAGE?

Quiescent lesions do not need treatment. Treat active lesions with a combination of systemic pyrimethamine and sulfamethoxazole; add folinic acid to prevent bone marrow suppression from pyrimethamine.

WHAT IS THE OUTCOME?

Depends on whether the disease is caught early. Once it is advanced, visual loss may be irreversible.

CHAPTER 67

Von Hippel–Lindau Disease

WHAT IS IT?

An autosomal dominant disorder marked by angiomas affecting the retina, cerebellum, and spinal cord, sometimes accompanied by polycystic lesions of the abdominal viscera and carcinoma of the kidney. Extraocular lesions are present in 25% of patients identified by their retina angiomas. About 50% of patients identified by extraocular lesions have retinal angiomas.

WHAT DOES IT LOOK LIKE?

Retinal angiomas are red or pink round masses typically located beyond the range of a direct ophthalmoscope in the peripheral retina. They have an enlarged feeder arteriole and draining vein. Some patients have a single angioma; others have several. Eventually the angioma leaks serum (hard exudates) that may creep into the fovea to disrupt vision. Severe leakage can cause retinal detachment.

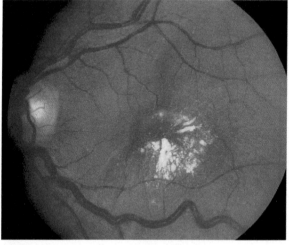

A

FIGURE 1. Von Hippel–Lindau disease. **A:** Hard exudates in the fovea reflect leakage from somewhere in the retina. *(continued)*

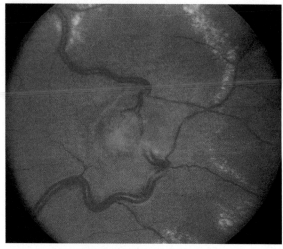

B

FIGURE 1. *Continued.* **B:** The culprit is a leaky, round, red lesion with feeding and draining vessels, a retinal angioma.

WHAT ELSE LOOKS LIKE IT?

Sickle retinopathy, peripheral retinal tumors. However, the enlarged feeding and draining vessels and the ringlike, hard exudates are not present in these mimickers.

HOW DO YOU DIAGNOSE?

By its characteristic appearance.

HOW DO YOU MANAGE?

All patients with retinal angiomas must undergo a systemic evaluation for extraocular lesions. Similarly, those with characteristic extraocular lesions should have ophthalmologic examinations to rule out retinal angiomas. The retinal angiomas are treated with intense photocoagulation or cryotherapy of the feeding arteriole.

WHAT IS THE OUTCOME?

Early identification of extraocular lesions may be life saving. Early treatment of the retinal angiomas is usually successful in obliterating them and preserving vision. When patients die of this condition, it is usually from complications of cerebellar hemangioma or renal cell carcinoma.

CHAPTER 68
Lysosomal Storage Disease

WHAT IS IT?

Metabolic dysfunction of lysosomes that leads to the accumulation of catabolic products within cells, which eventually kills them. Retinal findings may point the way to diagnosis.

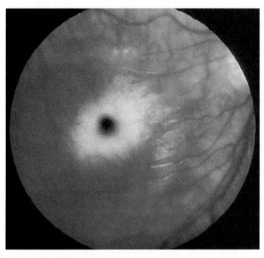

FIGURE 1. Lysosomal storage disease. This is Tay-Sachs disease, a gangliosidosis. Fundus photograph shows white halo around the fovea caused by opacification of retinal ganglion cells filled with ganglioside. Although this is a "cherry red spot," it is not caused by retinal ischemia as would be the case following central retinal artery occlusion (see Chapter 59). (as Photo courtesy of Wake Forest University Eye Center.)

WHAT DOES IT LOOK LIKE?

A cherry-red spot (gangliosidoses, sialidoses, Niemann-Pick disease Type A, multiple sulfatase deficiency, Farber's disease), bull's eye maculopathy, peripheral retinal pigment dispersion, attenuated retinal arterioles (Gaucher's disease, Niemann-Pick disease Type B, metachromatic leukodystrophy, ceroid lipofuscinoses, Hallervorden-Spatz disease, cystinosis), or optic disk pallor (Krabbe's disease, adrenoleukodystrophy).

149

WHAT ELSE LOOKS LIKE IT?

A cherry-red spot may occur in central retinal artery occlusion, but the history is that of acute visual loss in one eye. Bull's eye maculopathy may result from toxicity of chloroquine, hydroxychloroquine, deferoxamine, or thioridazine. Attenuated retinal vessels and pigment dispersion are nonspecific signs of widespread photoreceptor degeneration and are most commonly seen in hereditary enzymatic disorders. Optic disk pallor is a nonspecific sign of optic nerve damage. Bull's eye maculopathy, attenuated retinal vessels, retinal pigment dispersion, and optic disk pallor are also seen in nonlysosomal disorders such as peroxisomal disorders, spinocerebellar degenerations, mitochondrial disorders, and neuronal ceroid lipofuscinoses.

HOW DO YOU DIAGNOSE?

The retinal findings support the search for a variety of hereditary metabolic disorders affecting the central nervous system and not merely those caused by limited to lysosomal dysfunction. Therefore, a full battery of diagnostic tests must be run on such patients.

HOW DO YOU MANAGE?

Depends on the systemic diagnosis.

WHAT IS THE OUTCOME?

Depends on the systemic diagnosis. Some disorders can be slowed by appropriate management; the majority are untreatable at this time.

CHAPTER 69
Shaken Baby Syndrome

WHAT IS IT?

Trauma induced by rapid oscillation of the head. In most cases, the child is less than 12 months old. The oscillations cause shear injury of the brain axons as well as the subarachnoid and retinal surface vessels.

In young children, the jellylike vitreous has tight attachments to the retina. When the head is vigorously shaken, the retina and vitreous move at different velocities, placing stress on these attachments. As they tear, they rip holes in retinal surface vessels. Very severe injury causes tears within the retina as well. Retinal hemorrhages are present in more than 80% of cases of shaken baby syndrome.

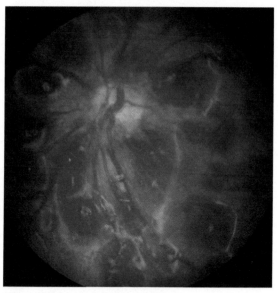

FIGURE 1. Shaken baby syndrome. Multiple large retinal hemorrhages reflect shear injury from shaking the baby's head.

WHAT DOES IT LOOK LIKE?

In mild trauma, one or more flame-shaped or round retinal hemorrhages appear at the interface between the retina and vitreous. In severe trauma, hemorrhages appear on, in, and under the retina, and the retina is thrown into folds.

WHAT ELSE LOOKS LIKE IT?

Severe coagulopathies or direct trauma to the eyes. Birth trauma, cardiopulmonary resuscitation, and a sudden increase in intracranial pressure can cause small retinal hemorrhages, but they are subtle and disappear within weeks.

HOW DO YOU DIAGNOSE?

The finding of a few retinal hemorrhages within the first month of life can be attributed to birth trauma. Persistent or extensive retinal hemorrhages, in the absence of a marked coagulopathy, are highly suggestive of shaken baby syndrome. Because nonretinal findings may be subtle, ophthalmoscopy is critical in making the diagnosis.

HOW DO YOU MANAGE?

Depends on the severity of the injuries. Child protective units assist in investigations leading to potential civil and criminal proceedings.

WHAT IS THE OUTCOME?

Depends on the severity of the injuries. Mild retinal hemorrhages usually resolve within months, often with full preservation of vision. More severe hemorrhages may lead to permanent vision loss.

CHAPTER 70
Retinopathy of Prematurity

WHAT IS IT?

Ischemic vasoocclusive and proliferative disease of the retina found in low-birth-weight infants. Infants at risk are those born at less than 36 weeks' gestation or with a birth weight of less than 2 g. Retinopathy occurs in 66% of infants with a birth weight of less than 1,250 g and in 82% of those with a birth weight of less than 1 g. At this stage, peripheral retinal vessels are still immature and stop growing if exposed to atmospheric oxygen levels. Fibrovascular membranes sprout from the areas of arrested growth, induce contracture of adjacent vitreous, and detach the retina.

WHAT DOES IT LOOK LIKE?

The retinal abnormalities occur in the periphery, well beyond the reach of a direct ophthalmoscope. A ridge develops between vascularized and nonvascularized retina. This stage may be followed by neovascularization and later retinal detachment.

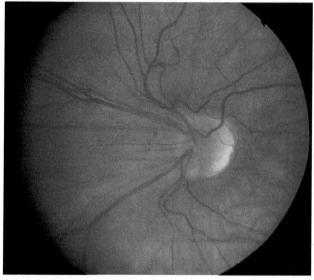

A

FIGURE 1. Retinopathy of prematurity. **A:** Dragged optic disk. A retinal fold distorts the optic disk. *(continued)*

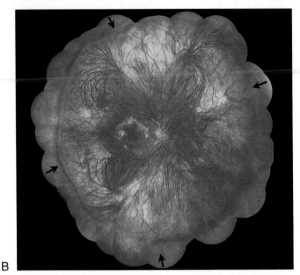

B

FIGURE 1. *Continued.* **B:** Peripheral shelf. In the retinal periphery, blood vessels stop prematurely and create a grayish circumferential mound. (Courtesy of Alan Frohlichstein, CRA, and Richard Hackel, CRA.)

WHAT ELSE LOOKS LIKE IT?

In an infant, these findings are specific. In older patients, sickle cell retinopathy, uveitis, and trauma might produce similar abnormalities.

HOW DO YOU DIAGNOSE?

By its characteristic appearance in a patient at risk.

HOW DO YOU MANAGE?

All children at risk should have oxygen monitoring and not be exposed to partial pressures of greater than 100 mm Hg. All suspects should undergo indirect ophthalmoscopy through widely dilated pupils either on discharge from the nursery or at 7 to 9 weeks of age, and again at age 6 months. A large controlled trial has shown that cryotherapy of moderately severe retinopathy significantly reduces unfavorable visual outcomes. Many ophthalmologists have found laser photocoagulation more effective than cryotherapy.

WHAT IS THE OUTCOME?

Spontaneous regression occurs in 85% of patients. Among those whose disease reaches moderately severe levels, cryotherapy or photocoagulation reduces the likelihood of blindness, but some children do not escape permanent vision loss.

CHAPTER 71

Retinoblastoma

WHAT IS IT?

A primitive neuroectodermal tumor arising in the retina. The most common intraocular tumor of early childhood, it has an incidence of 1 in 17,000 live births. It spreads locally to the optic nerve and meninges and metastatically first to the bone marrow. Untreated, it is fatal in a majority of cases. Curability depends on early diagnosis. Patients who have multiple tumors in one eye or tumors in both eyes have germ line mutations (chromosome 13q14) and a nearly 50% chance of passing on the tumor to offspring. Those with single tumors have only a 6% chance of transmitting the disease to offspring.

WHAT DOES IT LOOK LIKE?

A large tumor grows forward in the eye toward the back of the lens. When an ophthalmoscope light is directed through the pupil, the re-

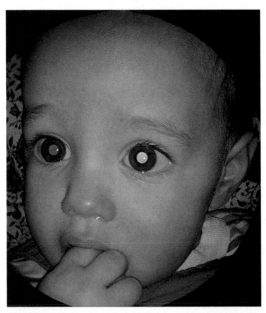

A

FIGURE 1. Retinoblastoma. **A:** Leukocoria ("cat's eye"). The left pupil looks white rather than the normal red-orange when an ophthalmoscope light is shined into it.

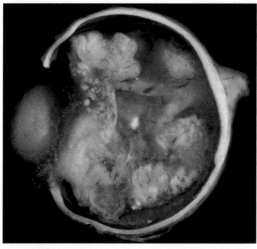

B

FIGURE 1. *Continued.* **B:** The cause of the leukocoria is a retinoblastoma that fills the enucleated eye shown here. (Courtesy of Wake Forest University Eye Center.)

flection is white instead of the normal red-orange (leukocoria). In other cases, retinoblastoma is detected when screening uncovers poor vision in one or both eyes or ocular misalignment.

WHAT ELSE LOOKS LIKE IT?

Leukocoria can also be caused by massive retinal detachment. However, the most common cause within the first 5 years of life is retinoblastoma.

HOW DO YOU DIAGNOSE?

Suspect retinoblastoma in an infant or young child if you find leukocoria. In the same age group, consider it as a possible cause of poor vision or ocular misalignment. A definitive diagnosis depends on a combination of ophthalmoscopy and imaging.

HOW DO YOU MANAGE?

Once a secure diagnosis has been made, ophthalmologists weigh several treatment options, including enucleation, radiation, photocoagulation, cryotherapy, and chemotherapy. The earlier the diagnosis, the greater the likelihood of saving vision and life.

WHAT IS THE OUTCOME?

Depends on the size of the tumors at diagnosis and whether they have already metastasized. With treatment, overall 20-year survival is 66%.

CHAPTER 72

Choroidal Melanoma

WHAT IS IT?

A malignancy of choroidal melanocytes. Nearly all patients are more than 50 years old. The tumor spreads locally into the retina and through the sclera into the orbit. The likelihood of distant metastasis, first to the liver, depends on tumor size at diagnosis and its cellular characteristics.

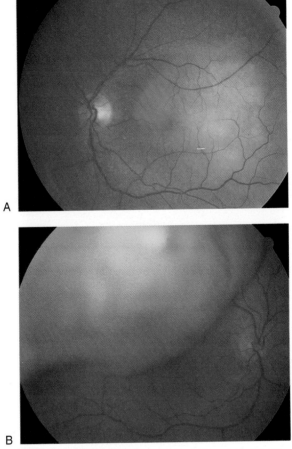

FIGURE 1. Choroidal melanoma. **A:** Brown subfoveal mass. **B:** Gigantic subretinal mass elevates the entire upper retina. *(continued)*

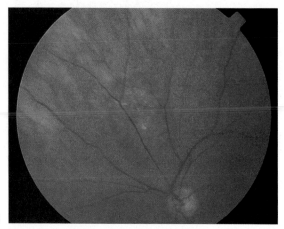

C

FIGURE 1. *Continued.* C: Small dark-brown lesion without mass effect easily mistaken for a choroidal nevus.

WHAT DOES IT LOOK LIKE?

A brown or black mound under the retina. Less commonly, the tumor may lack melanin and appear as a yellow-white mound. It may be discovered on routine ophthalmoscopy or if it distorts the retina and depresses vision.

WHAT ELSE LOOKS LIKE IT?

A choroidal nevus, inflammation, metastasis, hemangioma, hemorrhage associated with eye trauma, choroidal neovascular membranes in age-related macular degeneration, or choroidal inflammation.

HOW DO YOU DIAGNOSE?

By its clinical appearance, supplemented with history and the results of fluorescein angiography and ocular ultrasound, which yield a diagnostic accuracy of more than 95%.

HOW DO YOU MANAGE?

Optimal management remains uncertain. Most nonenlarging, flat, choroidal melanocytic masses measuring less than 2 mm in height are probably benign nevi and can be safely observed for growth. Large or growing masses are considered malignant, but a biopsy is rarely performed because of the risk of damaging vision or promoting metastasis. Before ocular therapy is considered, the patient must undergo a metastatic workup, including liver enzymes and chest and abdominal imaging. According to tradition, an eye bearing a suspected choroidal melanoma without evidence of distant metastasis should be surgically removed (enucleated). However, scleral plaque radiation is being explored as an alternative. Multicenter randomized trials are seeking the best way to prevent metastasis and preserve vision.

WHAT IS THE OUTCOME?

Depends on the size and cytologic features of the malignancy. Whether treatment is useful remains unsettled. Liver failure through metastasis is the usual cause of cancer death.

CHAPTER 73
Choroidal Metastasis

WHAT IS IT?

One or more metastases to the choroid. In men, carcinoma of the lung is the likely source; in women, carcinomas of the breast and lung are common sources.

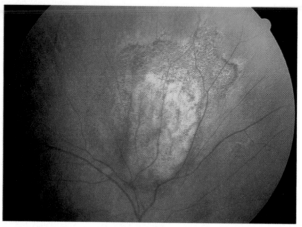

FIGURE 1. Choroidal metastasis. Yellow elevated lesion under the retina is metastatic breast cancer.

WHAT DOES IT LOOK LIKE?

One or more cream-colored masses hidden under the retina.

WHAT ELSE LOOKS LIKE IT?

Choroidal amelanotic melanoma, hemangioma. But these lesions do not grow as rapidly as metastases, and they are usually solitary.

HOW DO YOU DIAGNOSE?

By its characteristic clinical, ultrasonic, and angiographic appearance, together with the finding of a likely primary source.

HOW DO YOU MANAGE?

Once a presumptive diagnosis is made, the patient can be treated with local x-irradiation or systemic chemotherapy.

WHAT IS THE OUTCOME?

The lesions usually melt away within weeks of treatment, often leaving the eye with normal sight.

CHAPTER 74

Optic Disk Pallor

WHAT IS IT?

The neural rim of the optic disk appears gray-white rather than its normal orange-pink. This color change means that optic nerve axons have died and that visual acuity or the visual field is subnormal. But be aware of several important facts: (a) optic disk pallor can be very hard to appreciate, especially if it is binocular or if the ocular media are not perfectly clear; (b) many different conditions can cause it; and (c) it often lags weeks behind the onset of optic nerve malfunction.

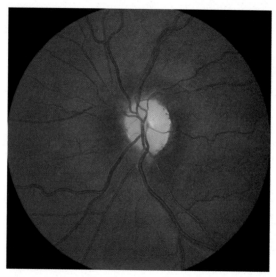

FIGURE 1. Optic disk pallor. The optic disk is white rather than the normal orange-red. This color change is caused by a loss of axons (from many causes).

WHAT DOES IT LOOK LIKE?

The optic disk rim appears gray-white instead of orange-pink. The color change may affect the entire rim or merely a segment.

WHAT ELSE LOOKS LIKE IT?

Normal optic disks often have relatively pale rims, especially on the temporal side. Tilted disks, especially those found in patients with high myopia, typically have pale temporal rims.

HOW DO YOU DIAGNOSE?

By the abnormal color of the disk rim. The color change is easier to appreciate if it is uniocular, by comparison to the normal fellow eye. Be careful not to overdiagnose optic disk pallor in eyes that have lens implants; removing the golden hue imparted by the aging crystalline lens makes the optic disk appear paler than in an eye that has a crystalline lens.

HOW DO YOU MANAGE?

Optic pallor implies optic nerve dysfunction. If there is no explanation, the patient requires an evaluation for various causes of optic neuropathy (inflammation; ischemia; hereditary, toxic, or nutritional disorders, compression by tumor).

WHAT IS THE OUTCOME?

Depends on the cause. Although dead optic nerve axons do not regenerate, vision sometimes improves when conditions underlying optic disk pallor are treated.

CHAPTER 75
Optic Disk Hypoplasia

WHAT IS IT?

Congenital deficiency of optic nerve axons. The common causes are congenital forebrain malformations and in utero infections or tumors.

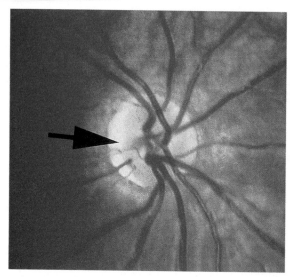

FIGURE 1. Optic disk hypoplasia. The disk diameter is abnormally small. The *arrow* marks the temporal disk margin; the white crescent is not part of the disk. This optic nerve is congenitally axon-poor.

WHAT DOES IT LOOK LIKE?

The optic disk is small. This condition can be hard to recognize ophthalmoscopically because the pale crescent that often surrounds a hypoplastic disk may be mistaken for part of the disk substance. Disk hypoplasia is easier to diagnose if it is uniocular and a comparison can be made with the normal eye.

WHAT ELSE LOOKS LIKE IT?

Nothing. The challenge is differentiating a hypoplastic disk from a normal one.

HOW DO YOU DIAGNOSE?

By recognizing that the disk diameter is absolutely small in relation to the size of its blood vessels and, where uniocular, relatively small by comparison to the normal disk in the fellow eye.

HOW DO YOU MANAGE?

Assume that this is a sign of maldevelopment, infection, or tumor of the diencephalon or other forebrain structures. Therefore, perform brain imaging and rule out hypothalamic endocrine dysfunction.

WHAT IS THE OUTCOME?

Depends on the condition. Hypoplastic optic nerves rarely allow normal vision, but it is unwise to predict how good vision will be in an infant because some mildly hypoplastic nerves allow normal visual acuity.

CHAPTER 76

Congenital Optic Disk Elevation

WHAT IS IT?

A congenitally full optic nerve head that forms a mound of tissue instead of lying flat within the retina. The elevation probably results from the fact that the optic nerve axons are crowded into a relatively small scleral opening. In most cases, the nerve functions normally.

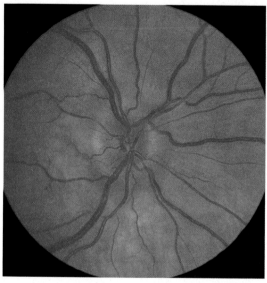

FIGURE 1. Congenital optic disk elevation. The margins of the disk are unclear, and it lacks a physiologic cup. A misdiagnosis of acquired optic disk elevation could be made, as in papilledema (see Chapter 77).

WHAT DOES IT LOOK LIKE?

The disk has blurred margins, and there is no physiologic cup. It may be tilted, and the branches of the central retinal artery and vein may emerge from an unusual angle. Sometimes yellow refractile clumps called drusen poke through the disk surface.

WHAT ELSE LOOKS LIKE IT?

Acquired disk elevation caused by increased intracranial pressure (ICP), inflammation, infarction, and neoplastic infiltration. Distinguishing between congenital and acquired disk elevation can be very difficult. Here are three clues: (a) cotton wool spots and disk surface hemorrhages do not occur in congenital disk elevation; (b) congenital disk elevation does not change its appearance over time; and (c) visual function is usually normal in congenital disk elevation and abnormal in acquired disk elevation.

HOW DO YOU DIAGNOSE?

By its characteristic and unchanging appearance, normal visual function, and the lack of historical features suggesting a process associated with acquired disk elevation.

HOW DO YOU MANAGE?

By serial examination to document lack of change in disk appearance and visual function.

WHAT IS THE OUTCOME?

Most patients with congenital disk elevation maintain normal vision. Some patients with optic disk drusen sustain slowly progressive visual field loss, but it rarely compromises visual acuity.

CHAPTER 77

Papilledema

WHAT IS IT?

Optic disk elevation caused by increased intracranial pressure (ICP). Papilledema lags behind ICP elevation, appearing several hours after a sudden rise and taking weeks to dissipate after the ICP has normalized.

WHAT DOES IT LOOK LIKE?

In early papilledema, the upper and lower disk margins become blurred. In more advanced papilledema, the entire disk margin becomes blurred and the disk rim rises. In very advanced papilledema, cotton wool spots and hemorrhages appear on a diffusely elevated hyperemic disk surface. In very longstanding (chronic) papilledema, a glial glaze develops on the disk surface. These changes are usually binocular, although they may be quite asymmetric in degree. Visual acuity is typically normal, even in marked papilledema. In the acute phase of papilledema, formal visual fields usually reveal deficits, but the patient is often unaware of them. In chronic papilledema, optic nerve axons may die in alarming numbers and severely compromise vision.

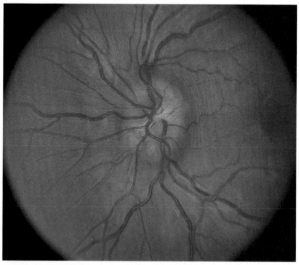

A

FIGURE 1. Papilledema. **A:** Mild. Disk margins are blurred.

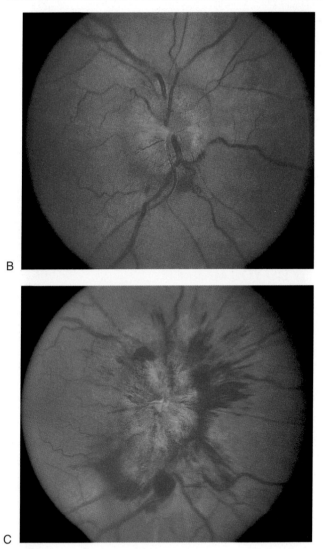

FIGURE 1. *Continued.* **B:** Moderate. Disk margins are blurred, and disk substance is elevated. **C:** Marked. Disk is elevated and covered with hemorrhages.

WHAT ELSE LOOKS LIKE IT?

Congenital optic disk elevation, optic neuritis, ischemic optic neuropathy, and neoplastic optic neuropathy. Early papilledema may be hard to distinguish from congenital optic disk elevation but not from the other acquired optic neuropathies, which usually impair visual function. Advanced papilledema is often confused with the other acquired optic neuropathies. However, for a given amount of swelling, the other acquired optic neuropathies usually cause far greater impairment of vision than does papilledema.

HOW DO YOU DIAGNOSE?

By finding disk margin blurring and disk elevation on ophthalmoscopy. Although papilledema may be hard to distinguish from congenital disk elevation, it is better to err on the side of overdiagnosing papilledema than dismissing it.

HOW DO YOU MANAGE?

By trying to lower the ICP through treatment of its underlying cause. If that cannot be done promptly, and the ICP remains markedly elevated, the optic nerves are at risk of ischemic damage. There are two surgical options: (a) cutting a hole in the intraorbital optic nerve sheath to allow cerebrospinal fluid (CSF) to drain out, and (b) shunting CSF into the peritoneal cavity via a catheter placed in a lateral brain ventricle or lumbar subarachnoid space.

WHAT IS THE OUTCOME?

The higher the ICP, the longer it lasts, and the weaker the perfusion of the optic nerve, the greater the chance of optic nerve damage.

Optic Neuritis

WHAT IS IT?

Inflammation of the optic nerve. It may be an isolated condition or be associated with multiple sclerosis (MS) or, less commonly, with a viral, bacterial, or fungal infection; connective tissue disease; or sarcoidosis.

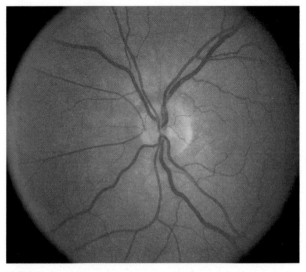

FIGURE 1. Optic neuritis. A normal optic disk is shown. Most patients with optic neuritis have no visible abnormalities of the optic disk. The process occurs behind the eye.

WHAT DOES IT LOOK LIKE?

The patient, usually between 10 and 50 years old, complains of acute or subacute loss of vision, typically in one eye and often accompanied by periocular pain aggravated by eye movement. Visual acuity may be normal, but the visual field is always abnormal. An afferent pupil defect is always present in the affected eye. The optic disk usually appears normal, although it may be swollen.

WHAT ELSE LOOKS LIKE IT?

Other conditions that cause acute or subacute optic neuropathy, such as compression by a retrobulbar mass, ischemia, or neoplastic infiltration.

HOW DO YOU DIAGNOSE?

By combining historical and ophthalmic findings with the results of ancillary testing such as brain imaging and lumbar puncture.

HOW DO YOU MANAGE?

Optic neuritis that is isolated or associated with MS is treated with intravenous methylprednisolone 1 g/day for 3 days, followed by a tapering course of prednisone for 11 days. Treatment hastens recovery but does not alter the outcome. Other forms of optic neuritis are treated according to the underlying process.

WHAT IS THE OUTCOME?

Depends on the cause of the optic neuritis. Patients with isolated and MS-associated optic neuritis usually recover fully or almost fully within weeks, with or without treatment. The visual outcome in other forms of optic neuritis is less predictable and depends on the nature of the process.

CHAPTER 79

Ischemic Optic Neuropathy

WHAT IS IT?

Infarction of the optic nerve. Most infarcts occur at the nerve head and cause optic disk swelling. The common causes are arteriosclerosis and sudden hypotension. But in patients more than 70 years old, suspect giant cell (temporal) arteritis, particularly if the patient has complained of a new headache, scalp tenderness, or pain on chewing (jaw claudication).

WHAT DOES IT LOOK LIKE?

The patient, usually more than 50 years old, complains of acute, painless loss of vision. Only one eye is typically affected, although in giant cell arteritis, the fellow optic disk may become infarcted within days if the patient is not treated. The optic disk is swollen. In severe infarction, it appears chalk-white because its blood supply has been extinguished.

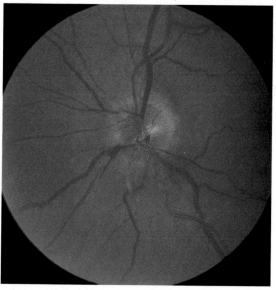

A

FIGURE 1. Ischemic optic neuropathy. **A:** Acute phase: The disk is edematous, primarily inferiorly. *(continued)*

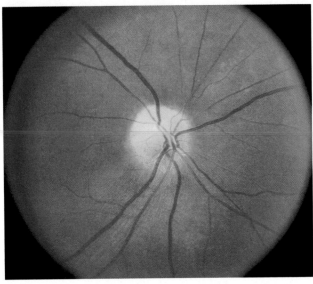

FIGURE 1. *Continued.* **B:** Chronic phase: In another patient, the superior disk substance has become pale (atrophic) where axons have died an ischemic death.

WHAT ELSE LOOKS LIKE IT?

Optic neuritis, neoplastic infiltration of the optic disk, and papilledema. Infarction is distinctive in being monocular, sudden, painless, and usually nonprogressive.

HOW DO YOU DIAGNOSE?

By combining historical and ophthalmic findings with ancillary studies, including laboratory studies aimed at diagnosing arteriosclerotic risk factors or systemic inflammation (erythrocyte sedimentation rate, C-reactive protein).

HOW DO YOU MANAGE?

There is no treatment for nonarteritic ischemic optic neuropathy. Discretionary arteriosclerotic risk factors must be abated. Patients suspected of having arteritic ischemic optic neuropathy should be treated immediately with high-dose corticosteroids (methylprednisolone 1 to 1.5 g/day i.v. for 3 to 5 days or prednisone 1.5 mg/kg). Within a week of commencing corticosteroid therapy, they should undergo temporal artery biopsy, which has a nearly 100% sensitivity to the diagnosis if performed and interpreted correctly. If giant cell arteritis is diagnosed pathologically, patients should be maintained for about 1 year on oral prednisone at the lowest doses that normalize acute-phase reactants and eliminate systemic symptoms.

WHAT IS THE OUTCOME?

Visual recovery is negligible. In nonarteritic ischemic optic neuropathy, visual loss may be mild and even preserve normal visual acuity. About 15% of patients suffer infarction in the fellow eye within 10 years. Whether arteriosclerotic risk factor abatement or oral platelet antiaggregants lower this risk is uncertain. The visual loss in arteritic ischemic optic neuropathy is usually profound. About 50% of untreated patients suffer infarction of the fellow eye within days to weeks. Prompt and intensive corticosteroid treatment reduces this risk substantially, but not to zero.

CHAPTER 80

Compressive and Infiltrative Optic Neuropathy

WHAT IS IT?

Compression or infiltration of the optic nerve by a tumor.

Compressive lesions—pituitary tumors, meningiomas, aneurysms, astrocytomas, craniopharyngiomas—usually lie near the optic chiasm. They typically cause slowly progressive visual loss in one or both eyes. An exception is hemorrhage within a pituitary tumor ("pituitary apoplexy"), which causes sudden visual loss. These tumors are generally visible on proper brain imaging.

Infiltrative neoplasms enter the optic nerve through the meninges. They are often invisible on imaging, but multiple lumbar punctures eventually detect malignant cells. Common sources are lung or breast carcinomas, non-Hodgkin's lymphomas, and skin melanomas. The primary tumor is usually found with a careful search.

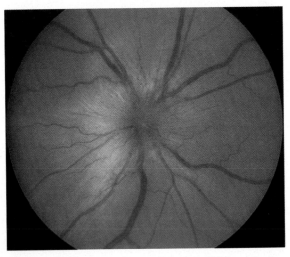

FIGURE 1. Infiltrative optic neuropathy. The optic disk is swollen because of infiltration by cancer.

WHAT DOES IT LOOK LIKE?

The patient complains of subacute and progressive visual loss in one or both eyes. Visual acuity or visual fields are always abnormal. The optic disks may appear normal, pale, or swollen. An afferent pupil defect is usually present.

WHAT ELSE LOOKS LIKE IT?

Optic neuritis, ischemic optic neuropathy, and papilledema.

HOW DO YOU DIAGNOSE?

By a combination of history, ophthalmic findings, and ancillary studies.

HOW DO YOU MANAGE?

Compressive lesions are managed according to the type of tumor. Meningeal cancers are treated with systemic corticosteroid therapy and x-irradiation; intrathecal chemotherapy may be considered.

WHAT IS THE OUTCOME?

With compressive optic neuropathy, visual outcome depends on the duration and intensity of compression. Decompression may restore normal vision. In infiltrative optic neuropathy, visual loss is often rapidly reversible, but the patient usually dies of metastatic cancer within 1 year.

CHAPTER 81

Glaucoma

WHAT IS IT?

Progressive death of optic nerve axons and excavation of the optic disk. In most cases, intraocular pressure (ICP) is pathologically elevated and causes or contributes to the optic nerve damage. The most common form of this condition, called primary open angle glaucoma, is of unknown cause. It affects about 3% of adults more than 40 years old. Patients at particular risk are African Americans and those with a family history of glaucoma or with high myopia.

WHAT DOES IT LOOK LIKE?

The patient does not appreciate any visual symptoms until the disease is far advanced. This is because visual field loss proceeds very slowly from the periphery toward the center. The optic disk always shows an enlarged cup. That is, the ratio between cup diameter and disk diameter is greater than 0.5. As the disease progresses, the inferior and superior portions of the disk rim become etched away. Eventually, the entire rim is lost.

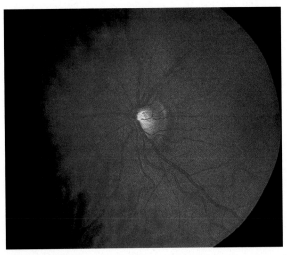

A

FIGURE 1. Glaucoma. **A:** Early glaucoma. The physiologic cup is vertically elongated because of some excavation of inferior rim tissue.

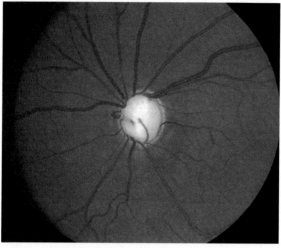

B

FIGURE 1. Continued. B: Advanced glaucoma. The rim tissue is almost completely excavated ("cupped out disk").

WHAT ELSE LOOKS LIKE IT?

Congenitally large optic disk cupping. This is a static anomaly. Rarely, acquired optic neuropathy caused by infarction, inflammation, or compression can produce pathologic disk cupping.

HOW DO YOU DIAGNOSE?

By a combination of optic disk cupping, characteristic visual field defects, and elevated ICP. In some cases, ICP is within normal limits.

HOW DO YOU MANAGE?

By lowering ICP when it is elevated. This is done with a variety of topical medications. If they fail, surgery is used to fashion a shunt (filtering procedure) between the anterior chamber and the subconjunctival space to allow aqueous to escape under low pressure.

WHAT IS THE OUTCOME?

In some cases, visual field loss and optic disk cupping are arrested or slowed down by treatment; in other cases, the disease progresses.

Anatomy

1. Eye—frontal view

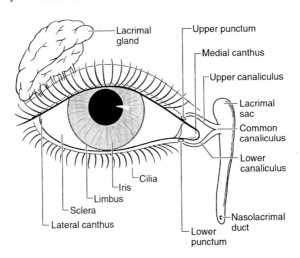

2. Eye—cross section

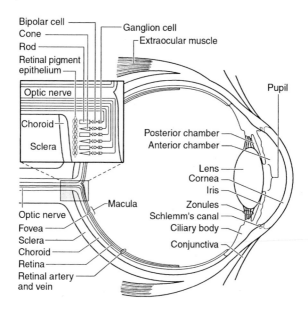

3. Eyelid

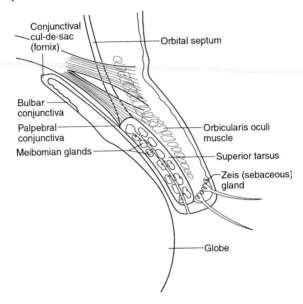

4. Orbit

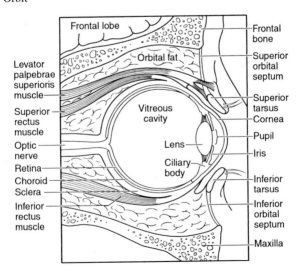

Screening Tests

Screening for eye disorders involves five main tests: (a) visual acuity, (b) visual fields, (c) pupils, (d) ocular motility and alignment, and (e) direct ophthalmoscopy.

VISUAL ACUITY

Distance Acuity

Measuring visual acuity on a Snellen chart placed at a distance of 20 ft from the patient is the most accurate method. In Snellen notation, the numerator designates the testing distance (20 ft or 6 m). The denominator is the number situated to the right of the smallest line of print that the patient can read. This number indicates how far away these letters would have to be before they would be just barely discernible to a person with normal sight. For example, a patient who is able to read no better than the 20/80 Snellen line is able to see at 20 ft what a person with normal acuity can see at 80 ft.

1. Test each eye separately with the customary glasses or contact lens correction used for distance viewing. For each eye, determine the smallest line of Snellen print that the patient can read. If most of the letters on a line are correctly identified, give the patient credit for that line.
2. If acuity is poorer than the largest Snellen letter (either 20/200 or 20/400), have the patient approach the chart as close as is neces-

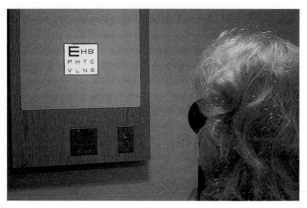

FIGURE 1. Distance Snellen visual acuity testing. The patient must identify letters on a Snellen chart at a distance of 20 ft (6 m).

sary to correctly read the largest symbol. If the viewing distance is 5 ft, record the acuity as 5/200 or 5/400, depending on the size of the largest symbol.

3. If the patient still cannot see the largest letter at a viewing distance of 3 ft, measure acuity by one of these methods, listed in order of decreasing visual function:

   a. Counting fingers: The patient can count fingers displayed at a distance of 1 ft.

   b. Hand movements: The patient can distinguish horizontal from vertical hand motions at 1 ft.

   c. Light perception: The patient can see a bright light shined directly into the eye.

Near Acuity

This test is used as a substitute for distance acuity when a Snellen chart is unavailable and to assess reading vision. It overestimates true distance acuity in uncorrected myopia and underestimates true distance acuity in uncorrected presbyopia.

1. Have the patient hold the near-vision card 14 in. from the eyes. (If you misestimate the test distance, the assessment will be inaccurate.) The patient's customary reading correction should be in place.

2. Measure acuity as you would using a Snellen chart.

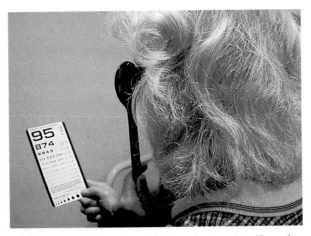

FIGURE 2. Near visual acuity testing. The patient must identify numbers from a Snellen near-vision card held at a distance of 14 in.

Qualitative Tests

When a patient is illiterate, mentally impaired, or mute, you must resort to qualitative tests of visual acuity.

1. Fixation and following: With one eye occluded at a time, observe if the patient's eyes stare (fixate) at a stationary target (a face, toy, or light) and pursue (follow) a moving target at arm's length. (This method is good for testing children aged 6 months to 3 years.)
2. Pictures: Ask the patient to identify standard pictures of diminishing size at a distance of 20 ft. Measurement is identical to that used in Snellen testing. (This method is good for testing children aged 2 to 5 years.)

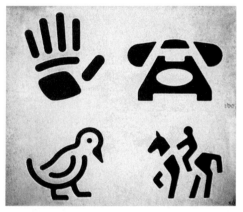

FIGURE 3. Picture acuity testing. The patient must identify standard pictures at a distance of 20 ft (6 m).

Normal Visual Acuity

Age	Normal Limits
6 months to 3 years	Ability to fix and follow a face, toy, or light
3 to 5 years	20/40 or better; one-line acuity difference between eyes
Older than 5 years	20/25 or better; no acuity difference between eyes

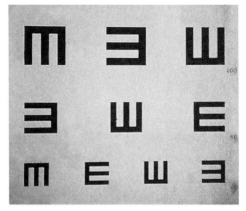

FIGURE 4. Tumbling E's: Ask the patient to identify (by hand gestures) the direction of the open portion of the three prongs of standard E's displayed in various orientations and sizes. (This method is good for children aged 2 to 5 years.)

VISUAL FIELDS

Whereas visual acuity testing assesses central (foveal, fixational) vision, visual field testing assesses peripheral vision. Highly sensitive and quantitative methods are available, but they demand time, expertise, and specialized equipment. The screening examination employs methods that usually detect only large or dense defects.

Drawing

The patient outlines defects on a piece of grid paper (Fig. 5). This method works only for small, dense defects close to fixation.

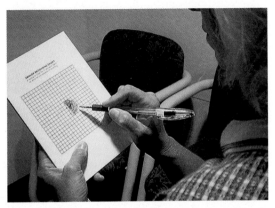

FIGURE 5. Grid. Patient drawing. The patient is asked to outline visual field defects on grid paper.

Confrontation

You display fingers, and the patient must indicate if he or she can identify them (Figs. 6 and 7).

1. Sit directly in front of the patient at a distance of 2 to 3 ft. Close your right eye and have the patient cover his left eye. Ask the patient to stare into your left eye. Check that your eye is positioned directly opposite the patient's eye. Position your hand in a plane midway between you and the patient. Instruct the patient to identify how many fingers you are displaying.
2. Display one or two fingers sequentially in each quadrant of the visual field (nasal superior and inferior, temporal superior and infe-

rior), approximately 10 in. from fixation. If the patient consistently fails to identify fingers in one or more quadrants, record this as an abnormality. If the patient correctly identifies fingers in all quadrants, move to the next step, which aims to detect more subtle deficits.

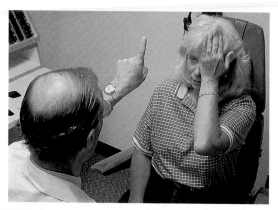

FIGURE 6. Confrontation visual field testing. Single-quadrant testing. The examiner displays one or two fingers in each quadrant as the patient fixes on the examiner's eye.

3. Display one or two fingers in two quadrants simultaneously, asking the patient to identify the total number seen. Always display

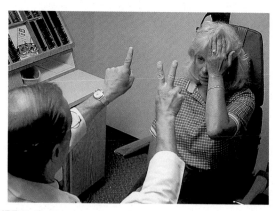

FIGURE 7. Double-quadrant testing. The examiner displays one or two fingers in two quadrants simultaneously.

two fingers in one hand and one finger in the other. Test the two superior quadrants and then the two inferior quadrants. If the patient consistently ignores fingers in one or more quadrants, record this as an abnormality. Repeat the same procedure with the patient's left eye viewing and the right eye covered.

PUPILS

The examination of pupils is aimed at discovering whether there is a lesion of the efferent limb (anisocoria) or afferent limb (afferent pupil defect) of the pupillary reflex arc.

Measuring Pupil Size in Dim Light

1. Have the patient fixate on a distant object in a darkened room.
2. Illuminate the pupils with a light from below the eyes, using the minimum amount of light needed to estimate pupil size.
3. Measure pupil diameter using the pupil gauge found on the near-vision card.

Measuring Pupil Response to Direct Light

1. Shine your light directly into the pupil of one eye, remembering to hold the light below the eye so the patient will not fixate on it (and cause pupil constriction to the near target rather than the light).
2. Note whether the pupil constricts strongly (rapidly and completely, or 3+ to 4+), weakly (slowly and incompletely, or 1+ to 2+), or not at all.
3. Repeat this test with the other eye.

Measuring an Afferent Pupil Defect

1. Have the patient fixate on a distant target in a darkened room.
2. Shine your light in the right eye as when measuring response to direct light (see above).
3. Swing your light across the nasal bridge so that it shines on the left eye. Note whether the left pupil constricts, dilates, or stays the same size. Normally, the pupil constricts slightly or stays the same size. If the pupil dilates, an afferent pupil defect is present in the left eye.
4. Swing your light back so that it shines on the right eye. A normal response is either slight constriction or no change in size.

5. Swing your light rhythmically back and forth between the patient's eyes to determine if there is consistent dilation of one pupil and constriction of the other. Consistent pupil dilation indicates an afferent pupil defect of that eye. Marked pupil constriction of the other eye is confirmatory. An afferent pupil defect strongly suggests an ipsilateral optic nerve or a severe retinal lesion.

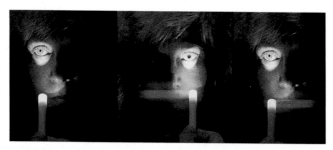

FIGURE 8. Afferent pupil defect. Testing for an afferent pupil defect. **Left:** The examiner shines a light onto the patient's face from below, assessing pupil constriction. **Center:** The examiner swings the light across the patient's face to shine into the left eye. In this case, the left pupil dilates, indicating a left afferent pupil defect. **Right:** The examiner swings the light back to shine into the patient's right eye, noting constriction of the right pupil, confirmation of a left afferent pupil defect.

OCULAR MOTILITY AND ALIGNMENT

In these tests, you are determining whether the eyes move normally and if they are in normal alignment.

Measuring Ocular Motility

1. Instruct the patient to follow your finger or penlight to the far right, far left, up, and down.
2. Decide if the amplitude of eye movements is normal. In right and left gaze, the white sclera should disappear into the canthus completely ("burying the sclera"). In upgaze, half the cornea should disappear behind the upper eyelid; in down gaze, two-thirds of the cornea should disappear behind the lower eyelid.
3. Decide if there is an ocular oscillation (nystagmus) in the extremes of gaze.

Measuring Ocular Alignment

1. Corneal light reflections test: Shine your light into the patient's eyes and note the position of the light reflections on the cornea. If the reflections are centered symmetrically, the eyes are aligned. If one image is outwardly displaced, the patient has a convergent misalignment, or esotropia. If one image is inwardly displaced, the patient has a divergent misalignment, or exotropia. If one image is upwardly or downwardly displaced, the patient has a vertical misalignment, or hypertropia.

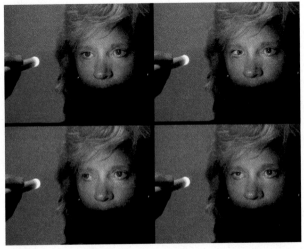

FIGURE 9. Light reflections. Corneal light reflections test for ocular alignment. **Upper left:** Normal ocular alignment. The light reflections appear symmetrically placed in the two eyes. **Upper right:** Esotropia. The light reflection from the inwardly deviated right eye is shifted outward. **Lower left:** Exotropia. The light reflection from the outwardly deviated right eye is shifted inward. **Lower right:** Right hypertropia. The light reflection from the upwardly deviated right eye is shifted downward.

2. Cover test:
   a. Have the patient fixate on an eye chart or object at 15 to 20 ft. For children, use a better attention-getting device such as a toy.
   b. Cover the right eye swiftly with your hand or an occluder and observe the left eye for a fixational movement.
   c. Uncover both eyes.

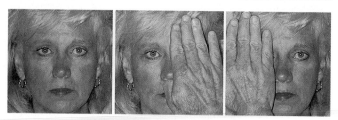

FIGURE 10. Cover test for ocular alignment: normal alignment. **Left:** The patient is fixating straight ahead. **Center:** The examiner's hand covers the left eye; there is no movement of the right eye. **Right:** The examiner's hand covers the right eye; there is no movement of the left eye.

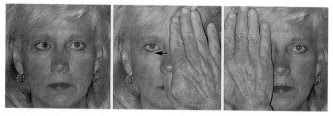

FIGURE 11. Cover test for ocular alignment: esotropia. **Left:** The patient is fixating straight ahead. **Center:** The examiner's hand covers the left eye; the right eye moves outward to fixate *(arrow).* **Right:** The examiner's hand covers the right eye; there is no movement of the left eye.

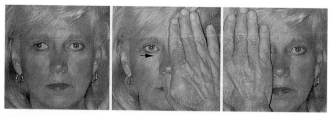

FIGURE 12. Cover test for ocular alignment: exotropia. **Left:** The patient is fixating straight ahead. **Center:** The examiner's hand covers the left eye; the right eye moves inward to fixate *(arrow).* **Right:** The examiner's hand covers the right eye; there is no movement of the left eye.

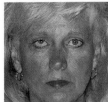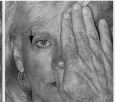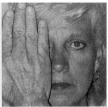

FIGURE 13. Cover test for ocular alignment: right hypertropia. **Left:** The patient is fixating straight ahead. **Center:** The examiner's hand covers the left eye; the right eye moves downward to fixate *(arrow)*. **Right:** The examiner's hand covers the right eye; there is no movement of the left eye.

   d. Cover the left eye and observe the right eye for a fixational movement.

   e. Determine alignment as follows: Lack of any movement in either eye signifies normal alignment. Outward movement of either eye when the opposite eye is covered signifies inward misalignment, or esotropia. Inward movement of either eye signifies outward misalignment, or exotropia. Upward or downward movement signifies vertical misalignment, or hypertropia.

OPHTHALMOSCOPY

Ophthalmologists examine the optic fundus with a variety of instruments, which allow a magnified view of the posterior pole and the retinal periphery. For screening purposes, the instrument of choice is a direct ophthalmoscope.

Looking through the undilated pupil provides a limited view even for those who have experience and skill. The recommended mydriatic agent for screening is phenylephrine 2.5% (2 drops instilled within 1 minute), a sympathomimetic drug that stimulates the iris dilator. Although weaker than the parasympatholytic drugs used by ophthalmologists (tropicamide, cyclopentolate), it produces adequate mydriasis within 15 minutes and lasts only about 2 hours. The risk of angle closure glaucoma is extremely low, and there are no other important side effects.

1. Select the ophthalmoscope's large-beam aperture and set its dioptric power to zero (Fig. 14).
2. Darken the room and have the patient fixate straight ahead on a distant target.
3. Position the ophthalmoscope so that its upper rim touches your upper orbital rim. Use your right eye to examine the patient's right eye, and your left eye to examine the patient's left eye. If you wear glasses, remove them.

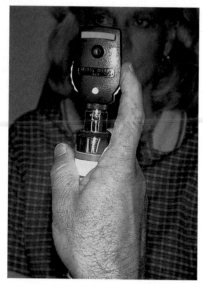

FIGURE 14. Holding the direct ophthalmoscope with the index finger on the dioptric dial initially set at zero.

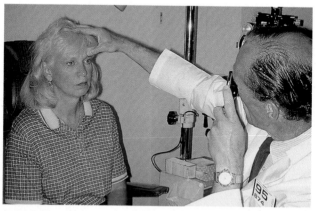

FIGURE 15. Examining for red reflexes. At arm's length from the patient, shine the ophthalmoscope beam into each pupil to see if there is a red-orange reflection indicating clear ocular media.

4. At a distance of 12 to 18 in. from the patient, shine the beam on one eye at a time, looking for the red-orange glow of the "red reflex" (Fig. 15). If you do not see it, the ocular media are not clear (or something is wrong with your technique so far). If the ocular media are not clear, do not expect to get a good view of the optic fundus.

5. If the pupils are not dilated, change the light aperture to small in order to get a better view of the fundus.

6. Place your free hand on the patient's head, your thumb elevating the upper lid and your four fingers positioned above the hairline (Fig. 16A). This helps in keeping the eye open and gives you a proprioceptive anchor as you approach the eye.

7. Approach the patient's eye gradually, aiming the beam 15 degrees nasally in order to view the optic disk. Bring the ophthalmoscope almost to the eyelashes, using your thumb as a guard (Fig. 16B). The closer you are, the better the view. If you notice obscuring reflections, reposition the beam so that it does not strike the iris. Dial the appropriate dioptric power to refine focus on the fundus.

8. Examine the optic disk for color, cup size, and margins.

Feature	Normal	Abnormal
Disk color	Pink	White
Cup size	≤One-half disk radius	>One-half disk radius
Disk margins	Flat, distinct	Raised, indistinct

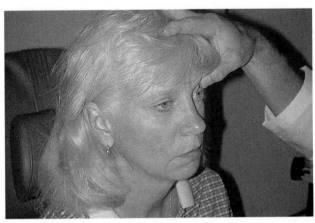

A

FIGURE 16. Examining the optic fundus. **A:** Position your free hand on the patient's scalp and retract the upper lid upward with your thumb. This maneuver keeps the lid open, offers proprioceptive guidance, and acts as a barrier to prevent your instrument from touching the eye. *(continued)*

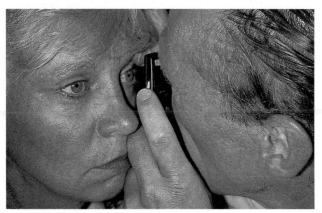

B

FIGURE 16. *Continued.* **B:** Approach the eye by aiming the beam 15 degrees nasally to hit the optic disk. The ophthalmoscope head should almost touch the patient's lashes. The thumb of your free hand acts as a barrier. Use your right eye to examine the patient's right eye, and your left eye to examine the patient's left eye (as shown here).

9. Examine the retinal vessels from the optic disk outward to their second bifurcation, looking for abnormal light reflections ("silver-wiring"), arteriovenous nicking, vascular sheathing, and intravascular yellow-white plaques.
10. Examine the nonvascular parts of the retina for hemorrhages, cotton wool spots (retinal microinfarcts), hard exudates (extravascular proteolipid deposits), and drusen (gray, round spots indicating the degeneration of retinal pigment epithelium).

Ophthalmic Procedures

INSTILLING EYEDROPS

Instilling eyedrops is not easy. Most drops end up on the skin. Here is how to avoid that:

1. Lean the patient's head back at least 30 degrees, making sure the patient is comfortable and gazing upward.
2. Hold the eyedropper bottle in your right hand.
3. Position the thumb of your left hand on the lash margin of the patient's upper lid and retract the lid upward, being sure you do not push inward on the eye, a maneuver that causes pain.
4. Retract the patient's lower lid with the fifth finger of your right hand, exposing the lower conjunctival fornix (cul-de-sac).
5. Release 1 drop into the fornix. *Do not release the drop directly onto the cornea and do not contaminate the dropper tip by bringing it into contact with the conjunctiva.*
6. Apply finger pressure to the nasolacrimal sac for 10 seconds to reduce systemic absorption.

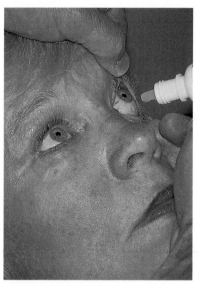

FIGURE 1. Instilling eyedrops. With the patient reclining, retract the upper lid with the thumb of your free hand and retract the lower lid with the fourth and fifth digits of the hand holding the dropper bottle.

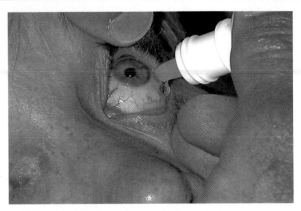

FIGURE 2. Releasing the drop into the lower fornix.

STAINING THE CORNEA

Corneal staining with fluorescein is useful whenever you suspect a defect in the corneal epithelium (trauma, dry eye, exposure).

1. Place a drop of topical anesthetic on the conjunctiva.
2. Wet a fluorescein strip with a drop of water and touch the tip to the inferior conjunctival fornix (cul-de-sac).
3. With a flashlight and magnifying loupe, or an ophthalmoscope set between +5 and +10 diopters, look for green patches or lines on the corneal surface that do not disapppear after blinking. These are defects in the corneal epithelium. They stand out even more clearly under cobalt-blue light (but not with a Woods' lamp).

EVERTING THE UPPER EYELID

Everting the upper eyelid is useful when you are looking for an airborne foreign body or severe allergic conjunctivitis.

1. Instruct the patient to look down.
2. Place a cotton-tipped applicator on the upper lid crease. Twirl it slightly in order to evert the upper lashes.
3. Grasp the lashes and pull the lid downward and outward, flipping it over the applicator, used as a fulcrum.
4. Use your thumb to keep the everted eyelid in place. The pretarsal sulcus mucosa will now be visible.
5. Inspect the pretarsal sulcus for foreign bodies (a loupe magnifier is helpful). If you find one, remove it with a moistened cotton-

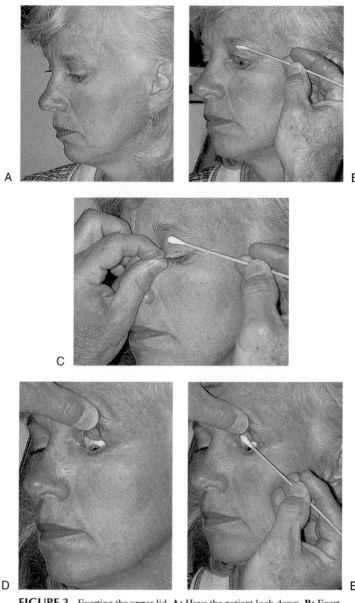

FIGURE 3. Everting the upper lid. **A:** Have the patient look down. **B:** Evert the lid with a cotton-tipped applicator placed at the upper border of the tarsal plate. **C:** Grasp the lashes with your free hand and pull the lid downward and outward (to break the seal between the lid and the eye). **D:** Fold the lid over the applicator, holding the everted lid in place with your thumb. **E:** Remove a foreign body from the superior tarsal sulcus with a wet cotton applicator.

tipped applicator, using a rolling motion. If you suspect allergic conjunctivitis, look for conjunctival mounds (papillae).

REMOVING A CORNEAL FOREIGN BODY

Corneal foreign bodies can often be removed with a moist cotton-tipped applicator. Slit lamp magnification is ideal, but a loupe will do.

1. Anesthetize the cornea topically and wait 1 minute.
2. Locate the foreign body (brown or black, transparent if glass) and attempt removal with a moistened cotton-tipped applicator. *Do not use needles or other sharp instruments unless you have considerable expertise and a slit lamp.*
3. If the epithelial defect is small (1 to 2 mm), no medications or patching is necessary. Instruct the patient to return for a reexamination in 24 hours if pain or blurred vision persists. For large defects, patching (see below) is helpful for comfort. Instillation of a topical antibiotic or cycloplegic is advisable. The patient must return for a follow-up visit within 24 to 48 hours.

PATCHING AND SHIELDING THE EYE

Patching is used to provide comfort when the cornea has been abraded. Shielding is used to protect the globe when you suspect that it has been lacerated or penetrated.

Patching

1. Place a single or double gauze pad over the closed lid and have the patient hold it in place.
2. Apply tape that extends from brow to cheek, making sure that the strips do not extend to the mandible (because opening the mouth will loosen the patch). Use enough tape to make the patch firm.

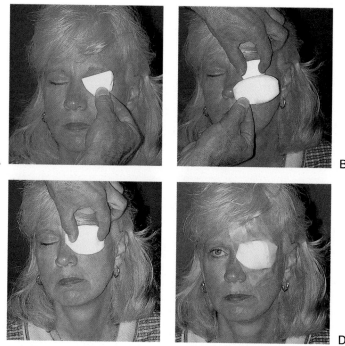

FIGURE 4. Patching. **A:** Fold a standard eye pad over the closed lids. **B,C:** Place an unfolded eye pad on top of the folded pad for extra bulk. **D:** Tape pads in place, making sure that the tape does not extend to the angle of the jaw.

Shielding

1. If a standard aluminum (Fox) shield is available, tape it in place. *Do not place any dressing underneath because there should be no pressure on the eye.*
2. If a standard shield is not available, cut off the bottom of a paper cup and tape as above.

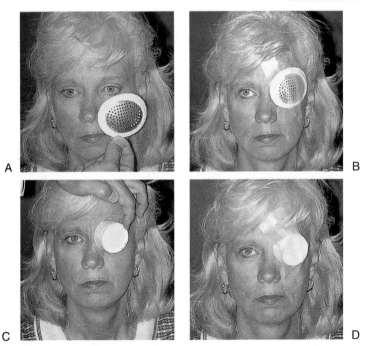

A

B

C

D

FIGURE 5. Shielding. **A,B:** Position a standard aluminum (Fox) shield so that its margins span the eye socket and tape it in place. **C,D:** If a standard shield is not available, cut off the bottom of a paper cup and tape it in place.

Managing Common Ophthalmic Problems

TRANSIENT VISUAL LOSS

Diagnosis

When the onset is abrupt, presume an ischemic mechanism (including migraine). When vision loss is not abrupt, the cause is less clear.

If the patient also describes flickering, flashing, zigzag, or shimmery lights, migraine is likely, especially if these scintillations last at least 15 minutes and appear restricted to one hemifield.

If the attack affects only one eye, presume ischemia to the eye; if binocular, presume ischemia to the visual cortex. *But it is very difficult to differentiate monocular from binocular transient visual loss because patients attribute hemianopic loss to the eye with the temporal field loss. One clue is that patients with monocular visual loss do not complain that their ability to read was compromised during the attack (one seeing eye is all they need).*

Although transient monocular visual loss is often attributed to emboli from the cervical vessels or heart, do not make that assumption without an eye examination to exclude papilledema or impending retinal vein, retinal artery, or optic nerve infarction. *Therefore, an ophthalmologic examination is a critical step in evaluation.*

Disposition

In monocular attacks in older individuals (age 40 and older), rule out carotid occlusive disease. Place patients on aspirin and have them evaluated promptly for an embolic source or a hypercoagulable state. Bear in mind that the likelihood of hemispheric stroke in patients with purely ocular ischemic symptoms who are treated with aspirin is less than one-half that of those who have anterior circulation hemispheric transient ischemic attacks (TIAs). Therefore, carotid endarterectomy is probably not indicated, especially in those who have medical conditions that aggravate the risks of surgery.

In monocular visual loss in younger individuals (less than age 40), an embolic source or hypercoagulable state is rarely found. They are presumed to have idiopathic vasospasm. However, an ophthalmologic examination, basic chemistries, and carotid ultrasound are warranted in order to make vasospasm a diagnosis of exclusion.

In binocular attacks, migraine is an acceptable diagnosis if there are scintillations that last at least 15 minutes. Otherwise, consider transient ischemia in the vertebrobasilar circuit. Patients older than age 40 should be evaluated for cardiac sources of emboli, arteriosclerosis, and hypercoagulable states. Carotid surgery is not indicated, even for high-grade carotid stenosis.

ACUTE PERSISTENT VISUAL LOSS

Diagnosis

Twelve conditions cause this symptom, three with red eye and pain (keratitis, acute angle closure glaucoma, and endophthalmitis) and nine without external signs (vitreous hemorrhage, retinal detachment, acute maculopathy, retinal artery occlusion, retinal vein occlusion, optic neuritis, ischemic optic neuropathy, occipital cortex infarction, and psychogenic visual loss). Diagnosis is difficult.

Disposition

Treat three conditions on-site and refer immediately:

1. Central retinal artery occlusion: Massage the globe with the index fingers of each hand (5 seconds pressure, 5 seconds release) 20 times in order to reduce its pressure. The low pressure may promote forward movement of an embolus or reopening of a thrombosed retinal artery. (Infusion of thrombolytic agents is still experimental.)
2. Acute angle closure glaucoma: Instill topical pilocarpine 2% every 5 minutes for three doses, topical timolol 0.5% one dose, and acetazolamide 500 mg one dose by mouth or vein.
3. Optic nerve infarction in giant cell arteritis: Immediately commence prednisone 2 mg/kg/day by mouth or methylprednisolone 250 mg every 6 hours by vein.

Refer three conditions immediately without on-site treatment: keratitis, endophthalmitis, and retinal detachment.

Refer the remaining six conditions within 24 to 48 hours (central retinal vein occlusion, optic neuritis, acute maculopathy, vitreous hemorrhage, occipital lobe infarction, and psychogenic visual loss).

DIPLOPIA

Diagnosis

Most diplopia results from misalignment of the eyes. It should then disappear when either eye is covered. Monocular diplopia, which persists when one eye is covered, is nearly always due to an optical aberration (cataract, uncorrected refractive error, presbyopia, keratopathy).

When diplopia is caused by ocular misalignment, the problem may be quite serious, especially if the symptom is recent. The lesion lies either in the central nervous system, ocular motor nerves, neuromuscular junction, or extraocular muscles. Localization depends on eliciting the history, measuring the misalignment pattern, detecting contributory signs (ptosis, pupillary abnormalities, proptosis), and obtaining the results of ancillary studies.

Disposition

Because management depends on the diagnosis, and diagnosis is often so difficult, new-onset diplopia should be handled promptly (within 24 to 48 hours) by an ophthalmologist or neuro-ophthalmologist.

FLASHES AND FLICKERS

Diagnosis

Flashes or flickers are visual hallucinations that come from the retina, optic nerve, or visual cortex.

Momentary white flashes in the peripheral field are often caused by an aging vitreous tugging or detaching from the retina. While this is usually a benign process, sometimes the detaching vitreous tears a hole in the retina, which could lead to retinal detachment, a surgical emergency. Therefore, new flashes in one eye demand prompt examination to rule out retinal detachment.

Persistent monocular flickers from one eye may reflect ischemic or inflammatory disease of the retina or optic nerve.

Binocular flashes and flickers always originate in the visual cortex. Migraine is the commonest cause, especially if the hallucinations consist of a zigzag sparkling line that expands across the hemifield over the course of 20 minutes. In migraine, the first episode of this hallucination may occur in late adulthood and without headache. The other causes of visual cortex hallucinations are focal epilepsy from a local lesion (tumor, stroke) or a posterior circulation TIA.

Disposition

If you suspect a retinal or optic nerve abnormality, refer for prompt ophthalmologic examination. If you suspect visual cortex discharge and cannot confidently diagnose migraine, refer for ophthalmologic or neurologic examination.

FLOATERS

Diagnosis

Floaters are black-gray spots, webs, or lines caused by particles in the vitreous cavity. Most commonly, they represent condensation of an aging vitreous. As the vitreous normally detaches from the retina in patients aged 60 and older, floaters suddenly appear. Other important causes are bleeding or inflammation in the vitreous.

Disposition

The new appearance of floaters should trigger prompt ophthalmologic examination to exclude retinal holes, detachment, hemorrhage, or inflammation.

DISTORTED VISION

Diagnosis

Persistent distorted vision, or metamorphopsia, is usually a monocular symptom and reflects edema or wrinkling of the fovea. Common causes are age-related macular degeneration, retinal surface wrinkling, trauma, and inflammation.

Transient distorted vision is a rare and usually binocular complaint that reflects inappropriate visual processing in the vision-related posterior hemispheric cortex. Common causes are stroke and tumor.

Disposition

Monocular metamorphopsia demands prompt ophthalmologic examination; binocular metamorphopsia demands either ophthalmologic or neurologic examination.

TEARING

Diagnosis

Tearing on cold, windy days is normal. Otherwise, tearing reflects overproduction or poor drainage of tears. Overproduction is usually caused by inflammation of the cornea, conjunctiva, or eyelids. Inadequate drainage comes from having poor apposition of the lower eyelid to the globe or an obstruction within the lacrimal drainage system (congenital nasolacrimal stenosis, inflammation, trauma, tumor).

Surprisingly, patients who have inadequate basic tear production from eyelid pathology complain of tearing. This is because their corneas dry out and stimulate reflex tearing from the lacrimal gland. The commonest cause is keratitis sicca, often a component of rheumatoid arthritis or Sjögren's syndrome.

Disposition

Refer any patient who complains of excessive tearing to an ophthalmologist. The urgency is greater if the patient also complains of a foreign body sensation, reduced vision, or periocular pain.

PAIN AROUND THE EYE

Diagnosis

Trigeminal irritation far behind the eye—as remote as the occipital meninges—causes referred pain in and around the eye.

Pain associated with a feeling of sand or gravel in the eye (a foreign body sensation) always reflects a corneal epithelial defect (trauma, drying, inflammation). Otherwise, periocular pain can be localized only within the trigeminal distribution, which includes the eye's surrounding soft tissues, the meninges above the tentorium cerebelli, and the cranial base blood vessels.

Disposition

One must hunt for structural abnormalities in the eye, its adnexa, and its cranial nerves. When the clinical examination is unrevealing, cranial imaging may be necessary. In some cases, such as cluster headache and trigeminal neuralgia, no structural abnormalities are found with any diagnostic studies. Periocular pain demands ophthalmologic examination. If the results are negative, a neurologic evaluation is indicated.

PTOSIS

Diagnosis

Ptosis, or drooping of the upper eyelid, may be caused by third cranial nerve palsy, Horner's syndrome, a neuromuscular junction transmission failure, or a levator palpebrae superioris musculotendinous disorder.

Third cranial nerve palsy is the urgent concern because of the threat of rupture of an aneurysm. When an aneurysm is the cause, other signs of third cranial nerve palsy (dilated, poorly reactive pupil; reduced ocular movement, ocular misalignment) are usually present.

Because the sympathetic pathway to the tiny Müller's muscle transverses the brainstem, spine, paraspinal region, chest, neck, and head, the lesion of Horner's syndrome may be hard to track down. The sympathetically innervated Müller's muscle makes a relatively small contribution to lid elevation, so that the ptosis of Horner's syndrome is always mild—never more than 2 mm. An important clue to Horner's syndrome is a smaller but reactive pupil on the affected side (miosis). (See next section, on Anisocoria.)

Myasthenia gravis, an autoimmune neuromuscular junction disorder, is a common cause of ptosis at any age. The ptosis typically fluctuates, being least prominent after sleep.

Ptosis may also be caused by musculotendinous disorders of the levator palpebrae of the upper eyelid. Congenital causes are common, and acquired causes include eyelid inflammation, chronic contact lens wear, certain myopathies, and degeneration owing to aging.

Disposition

Acute onset ptosis demands immediate evaluation by an ophthalmologist to rule out third cranial nerve palsy. Chronic ptosis should be evaluated nonemergently.

ANISOCORIA

Diagnosis

Anisocoria, or a difference in the diameter of the pupils, may be physiologic if the difference is less than 1 mm and both pupils react briskly and equally to light. Otherwise, it reflects a lesion in the parasympathetic or sympathetic innervation of the iris sphincter muscle or in the muscle itself.

Parasympathetic innervation failure causes a relatively dilated pupil that reacts sluggishly to direct light. The major concern, as with ptosis, is a third cranial nerve palsy, especially one caused by an aneurysm. However, isolated anisocoria is never caused by a third nerve palsy. Look for other signs of a third cranial nerve palsy (ptosis, reduced ocular movements, ocular misalignment). A common cause of isolated but permanent anisocoria is viral infection of the ciliary ganglion (Adie's syndrome).

Sympathetic innervation failure (Horner's syndrome) causes anisocoria in which the affected pupil is smaller, but both pupils react briskly to light. Ptosis is usually present but may be very mild. (See previous section, on Ptosis.)

Anisocoria is often caused by accidental (or even deliberate) instillation of parasympatholytic (atropinic) chemicals onto the conjunctiva or cornea. This occurs most commonly among hospital personnel and those exposed to atropine-containing plants.

Inflammation and trauma to the iris sphincter is another cause of anisocoria. The pupil is usually irregular in shape, and magnified examination shows evidence of muscle damage.

Disposition

Isolated anisocoria is rarely a cause for concern in adults. If recent diplopia or ptosis is present, evaluation becomes emergent. In children, anisocoria could represent Horner's syndrome caused by a neuroblastoma; evaluation is therefore more urgent.

Ophthalmic Medications

OCULAR ANESTHETICS

Examples
Proparacaine hydrochloride (Alcaine, Ophthaine, Ophthetic, AK-taine), tetracaine hydrochloride (Pontocaine, Anacel).

Effects
Anesthesia of the cornea and conjunctiva.

Ocular Side Effects
Damage to the corneal epithelium with chronic use. Therefore, *these drugs should never be prescribed.*

Systemic Side Effects
None.

Comments
Minimal discomfort with ocular instillation; onset of action within 1 minute, and duration 10 to 20 minutes. All preparations are equally effective.

MYDRIATICS AND CYCLOPLEGICS

Parasympatholytic agents paralyze the pupil sphincter (mydriasis) and ciliary muscle (cycloplegia). Sympathomimetic agents produce only moderate mydriasis and no cycloplegia. Mydriasis is used to obtain an improved view of the lens, vitreous, and optic fundus. Cycloplegia is used to reduce painful reactive ciliary muscle spasm in keratitis or uveitis and to suspend accommodation in order to obtain a more optimal refraction, especially in children.

Parasympatholytics

Examples
Tropicamide 0.5% and 1% (Mydriacyl), cyclopentolate 0.5%, 1%, and 2% (Cyclogyl), atropine 1/2%, 1%, and 3%.

Ocular Effects
Pupil dilation, loss of accommodation.

Ocular Side Effects
Angle closure glaucoma in patients with anatomically narrow anterior chamber angles. *This is very rare.*

Systemic Side Effects

Fever, skin flush, tachycardia, confusion (rare, predominantly in children treated with atropine or cyclopentolate); seizures (very rare, only in children with poorly controlled epilepsy).

Comments

Tropicamide is the most commonly used agent for ophthalmoscopy and refraction because of its brief duration of action (4 to 6 hours). Cyclopentolate and atropine are used for more complete cycloplegia in refracting children with strabismus and in treating uveitis. Do not use atropine for routine mydriasis or cycloplegia because of its extremely prolonged cycloplegia (1 to 2 weeks).

Sympathomimetics

Examples

Phenylephrine 2.5% and 10%.

Ocular Side Effects

None.

Systemic Side Effects

Phenylephrine 10% may rarely cause blood pressure elevation, cardiac arrhythmia, and myocardial infarction; phenylephrine 2.5% causes no systemic side effects.

Comments

Phenylephrine 2.5% is a useful agent to dilate the pupil slightly for direct ophthalmoscopy. But dilation is too weak to allow an ideal view. Duration of action is only 1 to 2 hours, and chances of precipitating angle closure glaucoma are negligible. Phenylephrine 10% should not be used because it may cause a severe rise in blood pressure, ventricular arrhythmias, and myocardial infarction, especially in patients being treated with systemic beta blockers.

ANTIBACTERIAL AGENTS

Sulfa

Examples

Sulfacetamide sodium 10% (many brands).

Ocular Side Effects

Allergic dermatitis of the eyelids (very rare).

Systemic Side Effects

Stevens-Johnson syndrome in patients previously allergic to systemic sulfa administration (very rare).

Comments

Good first choice for bacterial conjunctivitis, dacryocystitis, and blepharitis because it is inexpensive, is broad-spectrum, and has a low chance of side effects. Do not prescribe if the patient has a sulfa allergy.

Aminoglycosides

Examples

Neomycin, gentamicin, tobramycin (many brands); neomycin is often combined with polymyxin B and bacitracin to increase its spectrum of action.

Ocular Side Effects

Contact eyelid and facial dermatitis in about 10% of patients. This unpleasant side effect can be reversed with topical corticosteroids. Chronic ocular use of any aminoglycoside can cause keratitis.

Systemic Side Effects

None.

Comments

Together with quinolones, considered the most effective antiinfectives in treating bacterial conjunctivitis, bacterial keratitis, blepharitis, and dacryocystitis. However, gentamicin and tobramycin are expensive, and neomycin causes frequent contact dermatitis.

Erythromycin

Examples

Erythromycin ointment 0.5% (many brands).

Ocular Side Effects

None.

Systemic Side Effects

None.

Comments

Used primarily to treat neonatal inclusion (chlamydial) conjunctivitis, bacterial conjunctivitis, and blepharitis; relatively inexpensive and broad-spectrum, but available only as an ointment.

Quinolones

Examples

Ciprofloxacin (Ciloxan).

Ocular Side Effects

None.

Systemic Side Effects
None.

Comments
Potent, broad-spectrum, very expensive agents with poor streptococcal coverage.

Tetracycline

Examples
Tetracycline hydrochloride 1% (Achromycin).

Ocular Side Effects
None.

Systemic Side Effects
None.

Comments
Used primarily in prophylaxis of neonatal conjunctivitis.

Trimethoprim

Examples
Trimethoprim-polymyxin B (Polytrim).

Ocular Side Effects
None.

Systemic Side Effects
None.

Comments
Effective and broad-spectrum but very expensive.

Corticosteroid-Antibiotic Combinations

Topical ophthalmic combination corticosteroid-antibiotic preparations are prescribed as shotgun treatment for red eyes. The corticosteroid may eliminate the redness and pain, but an infection may proceed apace. The patient may not seek attention until the viruses or fungi have produced irrevocable damage. Therefore, *these combinations should be avoided.*

ANTIVIRAL AGENTS

Examples
Trifluorothymidine (Viroptic), vidarabine (Vira-A), idoxuridine, acyclovir (Zovirax); the first three are topical ocular agents; the fourth is available in the United States only for systemic administration, not for ocular application.

Ocular Side Effects
Epithelial keratopathy, conjunctival inflammation, and lacrimal punctal stenosis.

Systemic Side Effects
None.

Comments
Accelerates healing of herpes simplex keratitis. Acyclovir is used orally (800 mg 5×/day) to prevent severe keratitis and uveitis in patients with trigeminal herpes zoster.

VASOCONSTRICTORS AND ANTIHISTAMINES

Agents in these two classes, and combinations, are used to treat ocular allergy. They are often prescribed when systemic antihistamines fail to resolve ocular symptoms. Topical vasoconstrictors (naphazoline, oxymetazoline, tetrahydrozoline, phenylephrine) and vasoconstrictor–H-1 blocker combinations (naphazoline-pheniramine, naphazoline-antazoline) are available without a prescription. Stronger H-1 blockers (levocabastine HCl, emedastine, olopatadine) and mast cell stabilizers (cromolyn sodium, lodoxamide tromethamine, nedocromil, pemirolast) can be obtained only by prescription. An alternative is ketorolac, a topical nonsteroidal agent. If none of these agents adequately relieves allergic symptoms, topical corticosteroids may be necessary but should be prescribed by an ophthalmologist.

Vasoconstrictors

Examples
Naphazoline HCl 0.012%, 0.02%, 0.03%, 0.1% (many brands), oxymetazoline HCl 0.025% (Visine, OcuClear), phenylephrine HCl 0.12%, tetrahydrozoline HCl 0.05% (many brands).

Ocular Side Effects
Rebound conjunctival hyperemia.

Systemic Side Effects

May rarely cause hypertension and cardiac arrhythmia, especially in patients taking monoamine oxidase inhibitors or in those who have labile hypertension.

Comments

More effective for ocular allergy if used in combination with topical antihistamine (see next section). They should not be used to treat acute red eye without a definite diagnosis of allergy. Otherwise, they may mask a serious cause of inflammation such as keratitis, uveitis, or acute glaucoma.

Antihistamines

Examples

Pheniramine maleate 0.3%, antazoline phosphate 0.5% (many brands, usually in combination with naphazoline, a vasoconstrictor), levocabastine HCl 0.05% (Livostin), emedastine difumarate 0.05% (Emadine), olopatadine HCl 0.1% (Patanol), ketotifen fumarate 0.025% (Zaditen), nedocromil sodium 2% (Alocril), cromolyn sodium 4% (Crolom, Opticrom), lodoxamide tromethamine 0.1% (Alomide), pemirolast potassium 0.1% (Alamast).

Ocular Side Effects

Stinging on instillation.

Systemic Side Effects

None.

Comments

Well tolerated, but the powerful antihistamines are expensive and should not be prescribed for mild allergic conjunctivitis unless over-the-counter vasoconstrictor-antihistamine combinations have failed.

CORTICOSTEROIDS

Corticosteroids are the principal agents used in the treatment of ocular inflammatory disease.

Examples

Prednisolone acetate or sodium phosphate 1/8% and 1%, dexamethasone phosphate 0.1%, hydrocortisone acetate 0.2%, medrysone 1%, fluorometholone 0.1%, loteprednol etabonate 0.5% (Alrex, Lotemax), rimexolone 1% (Vexol) (many brands).

Ocular Side Effects

Dose-dependent elevation in intraocular pressure (ICP) that is usually reversible on stopping the drug.

Systemic Side Effects

None.

Comments

Potentially dangerous if an infection has not been excluded, especially in an immunocompromised host, a possibly ruptured globe, ocular trauma involving plants or soil, or chronic treatment of a red eye. Avoid combinations of corticosteroids and antiinfectives as shotgun therapy.

ARTIFICIAL TEAR PREPARATIONS

Artificial tear preparations replace natural tears in tear-deficiency states (Sjögren's syndrome, ocular pemphigoid, ocular radiation, and chemical burn) and prolong tear contact with the cornea when it is abnormally exposed (seventh cranial nerve palsy, ectropion).

Polyvinyl alcohol preparations are the least viscous, followed by cellulose ester preparations. Among the latter, the most viscous are carboxymethylcellulose preparations (Celluvisc, Refresh Plus, Thera Tears). For patients with severely dry or exposed eyes, viscous preparations are more effective. For such conditions, petrolatum-based ointments (Duratears Naturale, LubriTears, HypoTears, Lacri-Lube, Refresh PM), usually instilled before bedtime, are options. Ointments are not popular for daytime use because they are uncomfortable and blur vision.

Many patients develop pain and conjunctival inflammation from allergies to the preservatives in artificial tears. For such individuals, tears are available in preservative-free (and very costly), single-dose vials.

Cellulose Esters

Examples

Hydroxy ethylcellulose, hydroxypropyl cellulose, hydroxypropyl methylcellulose, methylcellulose, carboxymethylcellulose.

Ocular Side Effects

Blurred vision and sticky lids from increased tear viscosity.

Systemic Side Effects

None.

Comments

Inexpensive, but efficacy is limited by the short duration of action.

Polyvinyl Alcohol

Examples
Polyvinyl alcohol.

Ocular Side Effects
None.

Systemic Side Effects
None

Comments
Often preferred over cellulose esters by patients because it is less viscous, but it is limited by the short duration of action.

GLAUCOMA AGENTS

Medications used to treat glaucoma aim to control intraocular pressure by reducing the production of aqueous humor or by increasing its outflow. Four classes of antiglaucoma medications, all administered topically, act directly on the autonomic nervous system. Absorption into the systemic circulation puts patients at risk for potentially serious systemic side effects. One class of antiglaucoma drugs, administered topically or systemically, inhibits the formation of aqueous humor by blocking carbonic anhydrase in the ciliary epithelium. The systemically administered carbonic anhydrase inhibitors cause important systemic side effects.

Adrenergic Agonists

Examples
Epinephrine (Epifrin) and dipivefrin (Propine).

Ocular Side Effects
Conjunctival hyperemia, black conjunctival deposits (drug metabolites).

Systemic Side Effects
Uncommon, but include tachycardia, premature ventricular contractions, hypertension, tremor, anxiety.

Comments
Used in conjunction with other antiglaucoma drugs; reasonably well tolerated, but they are of relatively low potency and may cause important ocular and systemic side effects.

Alpha-2 Adrenergic Agonists

Examples
Apraclonidine HCl 0.5% (Iopidine), brimonidine tartrate 0.2% (Alphagan).

Ocular Side Effects
Allergic conjunctivitis.

Systemic Side Effects
None.

Comments
Mildly effective agents used mainly as adjuncts.

Beta Adrenergic Antagonists

Examples
Timolol (Timoptic), betaxolol (Betoptic R), levobunolol (Betagan R), carteolol HCl (Ocupress).

Ocular Side Effects
None.

Systemic Side Effects
Bradycardia, reduced cardiac output and exercise tolerance, bronchospasm, hypotension and syncope, reduced libido, lethargy, and depression.

Comments
Because they cause no ocular side effects, beta-adrenergic antagonists are frequently prescribed. But their systemic side effects may be dangerous.

Cholinergic Agonists

Examples
Pilocarpine (many brands).

Ocular Side Effects
Pupil constriction, conjunctival hyperemia, brow ache or headache and, in younger patients, ciliary spasm causing myopia.

Systemic Side Effects
Patients who overdose (1 drop/hour) may experience cholinergic effects such as abdominal cramping, vomiting, diarrhea, diaphoresis, and bronchospasm.

Comments
Inexpensive and effective, but ocular side effects limit use.

Carbonic Anhydrase Inhibitors (CAIs)

Examples
Acetazolamide (Diamox), dichlorphenamide (Daranide), methazolamide (Neptazane), dorzolamide HCl (Trusopt), brinzolamide 1% (Azopt), dorzolamide HCl 2% and timolol maleate 0.5% (Cosopt).

Ocular Side Effects
None.

Systemic Side Effects
Topically administered agents (dorzolamide, brinzolamide) have few systemic side effects; systemically administered agents (acetazolamide, dichlorphenamide, methazolamide) have the following important side effects:

1. Stevens-Johnson syndrome (erythema multiforme) and blood dyscrasias. Both side effects are idiosyncratic allergic reactions. Stevens-Johnson syndrome is prevalent among sulfa-allergic patients. Blood dyscrasias, particularly aplastic anemia, generally occur within the first 6 months of drug use and tend to be reversed as soon as therapy is stopped. Between 1972 and 1984, 79 allergic reactions to CAIs were reported to the National Registry of Drug-Induced Ocular Side Effects; one-third were fatal.
2. Renal stones associated with long-term CAI therapy. Patients should be advised to avoid dehydration.
3. Paresthesias of the hands and feet and abnormal taste sensation (dysgeusia) are immediate effects that usually become tolerable with prolonged use
4. Anorexia, lassitude, loss of libido, and impotence are less prevalent and insidious. They may go unreported but can be very debilitating.
5. Systemic acidosis may develop during the first 2 weeks secondary to potassium and bicarbonate diuresis. These effects are self-limited and are usually not dangerous unless a patient is already potassium-depleted from either thiazide use or renal disease.

Comments
The systemic side effects have limited the utility of systemically administered CAIs. Topically administered CAIs have eliminated this problem, but they are less potent in lowering ICP. Patients placed on systemic CAIs should have periodic blood counts during the first year of treatment. To prevent renal stones, they should avoid dehydration. Supplemental potassium and calcium may attenuate the nausea and lassitude.

Prostaglandin Analogs

Examples
Latanoprost 0.05% (Xalatan).

Ocular Side Effects
Blue irides may turn brown, an irreversible effect (20%); uveitis, macular edema (rare).

Systemic Side Effects
None.

Comments
This agent has become very popular because it lacks serious ocular or systemic side effects and is effective in lowering the ICP. But it is very expensive.

REFERENCE

Trobe JD: *The Physician's Guide to Eye Care*. American Academy of Ophthalmology, San Francisco, 2001.

Subject Index

Page numbers followed by *f* refer to figures